FINDING
YOUR FEET

CONWAY
Bloomsbury Publishing Plc
50 Bedford Square, London, WC1B 3DP, UK
29 Earlsfort Terrace, Dublin 2, Ireland

To find out more about our authors and books visit
www.bloomsbury.com and sign up for our newsletters

FINDING YOUR FEET

The how-to guide to hiking and adventuring

Rhiane Fatinikun MBE

CONWAY

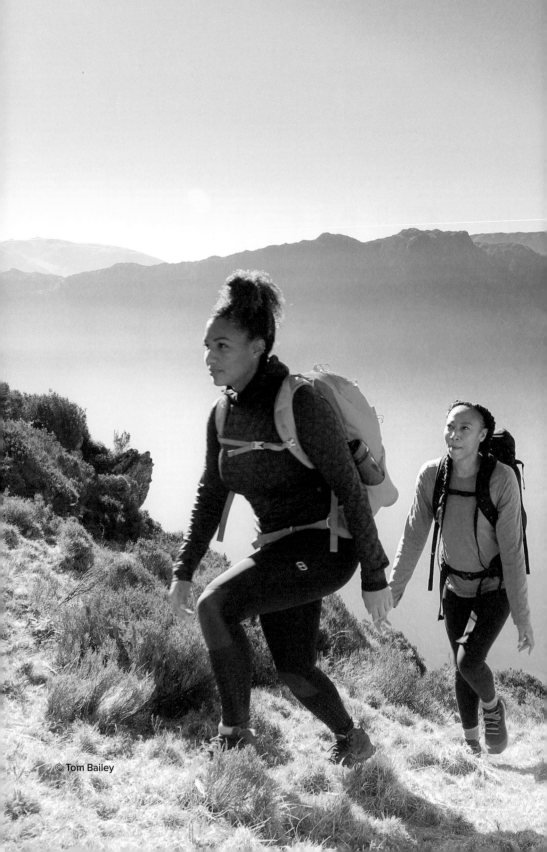

© Tom Bailey

CONTENTS

PART 2: HOW? 74

PART 3: WHERE? 120

INTRODUCTION

Welcome *to Finding Your Feet: The how-to guide to hiking and adventuring.* This is a book I have wanted to write for a long time, almost since that first day in 2019 when I resolved to take up hiking while travelling by train through the beautiful Peak District. I asked for buddies to accompany me on my hikes, which led to me setting up Black Girls Hike (BGH). And what started as a walk for a few women in my local area has become a national organisation with thousands of members. I also want to share how deepening my relationship with the natural world has transformed my life. Not only has it greatly improved my mental and physical health, but it has given me a new career.

Though BGH was started to provide a safe, inclusive space for women to explore the countryside, it has become so much more. For its members, it is a support system, a sisterhood where we can just 'be'. Many of us live with the pressure of constant code-switching, often being 'the only one' in our working lives. In the outdoors, among people who like look us, BGH provides a place to breathe. But this is just the start.

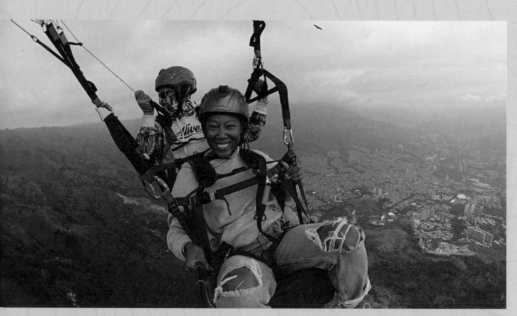

➡ Paragliding over Medellín, Columbia. A world of adventure awaits!

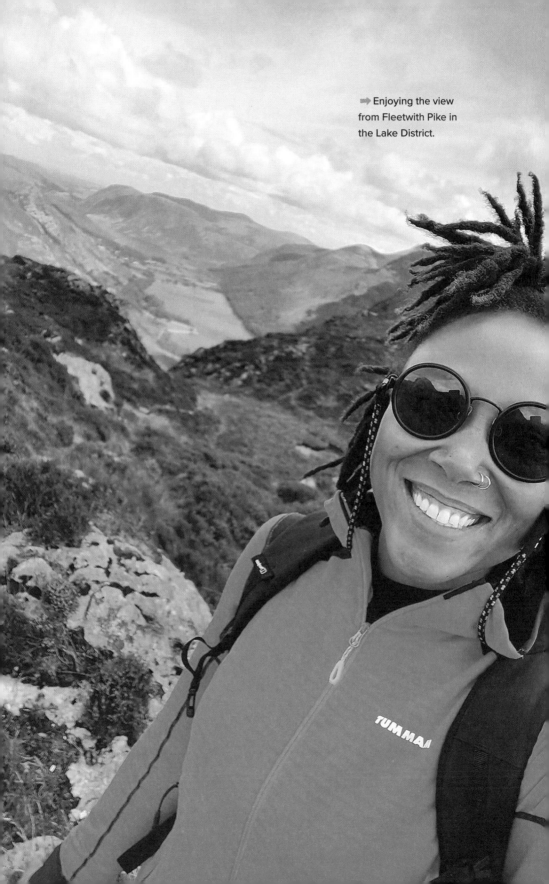

Enjoying the view from Fleetwith Pike in the Lake District.

One of the key aims in my work is to encourage and motivate more women who don't yet have the confidence to explore the great outdoors to do just that. *Everybody* has the right to enjoy the beautiful countryside the UK has to offer. It is my passion and my joy, and I hope this book helps it to become yours too. I want to show you that the countryside can be welcoming and inspiring. For not only is spending time in nature excellent for your physical well-being, but it also gives you a mental boost.

In the pages that follow you'll find all the advice I wish I had been given when I took my first steps into the world of adventure. All of it is practical, jargon-free and achievable. So I have included a guide to the kit you actually need (and it's less expensive than you think!), basic map-reading skills, how to be a responsible hiker, as well as some of my favourite routes to try. Throughout there are interviews with some wonderful women I have met on my journey who themselves have taken a leap and embraced the natural world. They are funny, honest, and truly inspiring. I can't wait for you to meet them!

I have also written here about my own journey from desk-bound civil servant to full-time adventurer. I've come a long way, very quickly. By sharing my journey, I want to inspire women to enjoy the truly amazing benefits the natural world has to offer. I truly believe that it doesn't matter if you are conquering a mountain range, completing a cliff-top ramble or exploring the green spaces on your doorstep, the health advantages are the same: a calmer mind and fitter body await! Willingness is what's important here – all you need to start becoming a hiker is to put one foot in front of the other. This is exactly how I started. And who knows where those first

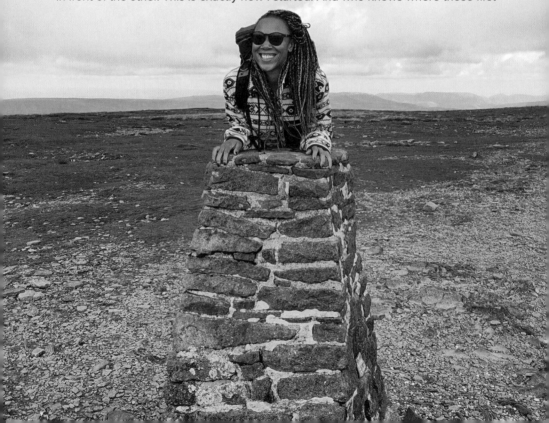

WHEN DOES A WALK BECOME A HIKE?

Speaking of hikes, you might wonder, *When does a walk become a hike?* That's up to you! Generally speaking, a hike takes place in natural or wild environments (so not in an urban one, though 'urban hikes' are actually growing in popularity). This book is called *Finding Your Feet* because, when I embraced the lush beauty of the natural world, I literally found my feet.

I discovered not only a hobby, but my purpose. My new career has fed my soul like nothing before. Now, as well as organising adventures all over the world and running a national organisation, I work full time encouraging minoritised people to do the same. My greatest pleasure is seeing how exposure to the natural world has benefited so many of our BGH members and the other groups we work with. Some of our brilliant regional group leaders have trained to be guides, and you will also find some of their wonderful stories inside. I am so proud of them and I now want to spread the BGH message to all women.

steps might lead? Five years ago, I would never have dreamt I would be kayaking Norwegian fjords or leading hikes across Ghana.

There are so many reasons to get outside. Maybe you have always wanted to explore the countryside but are afraid it will be unwelcoming or feel uncomfortable. Or you started walking during the Covid-19 pandemic but, with the return to everyday life, have since lost touch with nature because you no longer have the time or motivation to walk every day. Perhaps you want to get a new perspective on your own country, and have too often felt like a visitor rather than a resident. This book is written for you because I was you a few short years ago.

If you already regularly enjoy being in nature, and want to join a growing band of committed hikers. You can use the advice in this book to step up to the next level of adventure: more challenging routes, longer hikes or new activities. I've included a selection of my favourite walks, but also advice about hiking over a weekend, or for an even longer, epic hike on one of the National Trails which criss-cross the country.

Believe me, you have nothing to lose and everything to gain. Your relationship with the natural world will become central to your life and will have a positive impact every single day. You can look forward to a closer relationship with your environment, experiencing the changes in the seasons in a new, intense way, learning to recognise birdcalls, or simply observing how the trees change with the seasons.

New friends await you on this journey; inspiring and brave women who have your back. Wilderness is out there waiting for you. Take a step into the unknown. It will be worth it, I promise.

LOTS OF LOVE

Rhiane

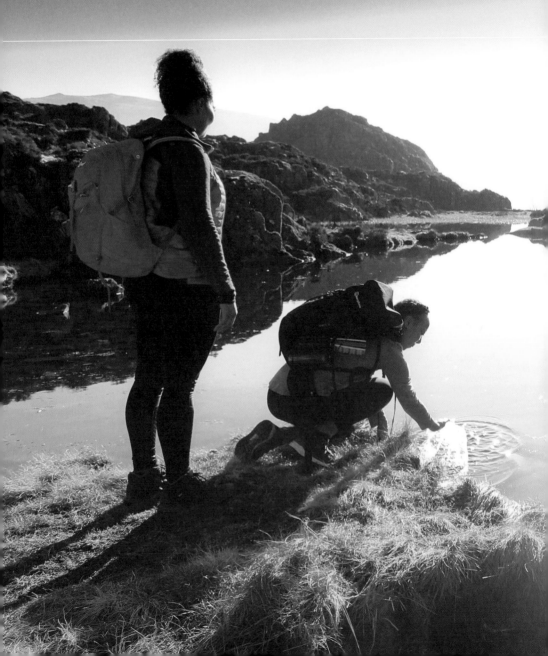

PART 1

WHY?

This book aims to give you all the information you need to help you start your outdoor adventure. It is also the story of how I re-started my life and found a career in nature. I wasn't born into an 'outdoorsy' family, and I had an office job until my mid-thirties – so the experiences I relate here are to show that anyone can stride out into the countryside. My story owes a lot to chance – it's all happened without a masterplan, but it also took a great deal of hard work and commitment!

But sometimes inspiration just isn't enough, and you need other people's practical advice. So, along with my life story, there are interviews here with women who have stepped out of their comfort zones (and sometimes their jobs and homes!) to achieve their dreams. They tell you honestly how they progressed in the outdoor world, whether this was a new hobby, a new career or simply a closer bond with nature.

Of course, when I set up Black Girls Hike, it was because I wanted a community to go out on hikes with. I didn't realise then that I would be bringing together a truly impressive group of outdoor enthusiasts who would go on to make BGH the organisation it is today.

These are some of the women I have met along the way. They are adventurous, courageous, and really embody the BGH ethos. As leaders, environmentalists and enthusiasts these women represent the community that, prior to 2019, I didn't know existed.

BGH women lift each other up, and through BGH training, projects and advocacy they embody a more inclusive future, for both participating in adventure and the professional profile of the outdoor industries. They are of various ages and backgrounds, and I am very proud of them. I hope you enjoy their stories.

MY STORY

My journey into an outdoor life was one of chance: I decided to go hiking, looked for buddies, and before I knew it was featured on national TV programmes and giving quotes to newspapers! In what follows I want to share some of the lessons I have learned along the way, and how I responded by drawing on my internal resources. It is organised under these headings, so you can focus on the sections which address those areas where you feel you need a boost, whether it is more courage, more tenacity or another quality.

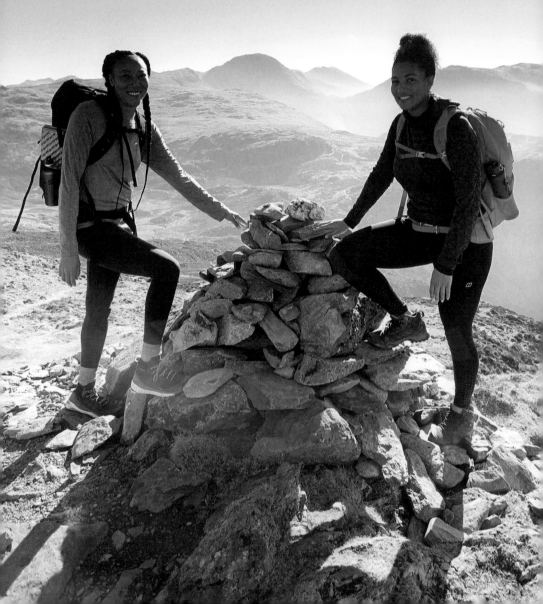

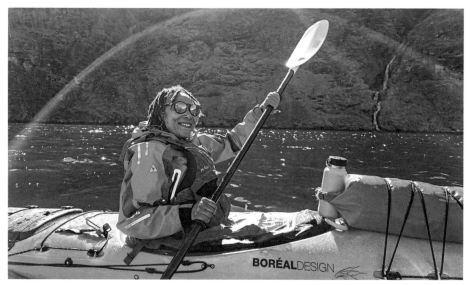

➡ ABOVE: Kayaking in Norway.
➡ LEFT: Ingleborough Trig in the Yorkshire Dales. © Tom Bailey

STRENGTH

My school years were OK. Education was really important in my family and they had high expectations of me academically. In high school, I was in the top set for everything, but when it came to the next step, I found that I hated higher education. In the end I made three attempts at getting a degree. At the University of Nottingham, I studied sociology and cultural studies, and at the University of Birmingham, I did public relations and business management. I didn't take to either course, but I did enjoy myself. I was always ready to party! Then, eight years later, I started doing international studies with the Open University. But I was working by then, and volunteering, and doing that alongside a degree was overwhelming. I just had too much on my plate alongside a full-time

job. I went to one seminar in four years and ended up cramming at the end of every month just to get through.

One night, after rushing through another piece of coursework at gone midnight to make a deadline, and knowing I had a full day of work ahead of me, I thought to myself, *What am I doing? I'm just pressuring myself because I want to have a degree.* I didn't feel like I was learning anything. My schedule and workload had become too stressful, and by setting myself this goal I felt like I'd put myself in a prison. After that night, I began to see things differently. I asked myself, *Who am I doing this for? I feel this is something that I have to do, but no one's forcing me. It's all in my mind.* In the end, I was so relieved when I gave it up.

I'm over it now and today I have

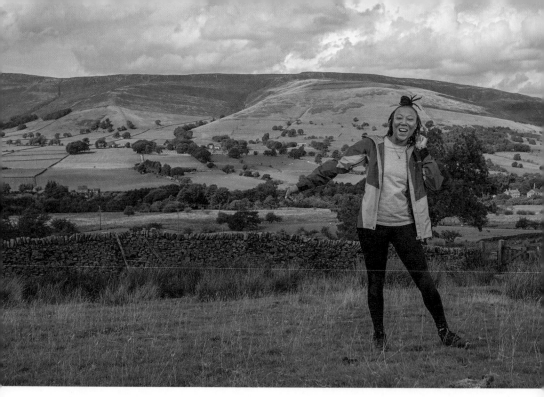

➡ I began my hiking adventures in the beautiful Peak District.

found different ways of measuring my achievements, but as I advanced through my twenties I started to feel in limbo. I thought that, unlike my peers, I wasn't meeting milestones in life. I had an office job, but they had careers. I hadn't set myself strong foundations for the rest of my life.

First, I had a job in recruitment, then one in social housing. After that, I started to work at the civil service but even when I became the union representative for my workplace and volunteered with community-based organisations (and in addition to all this started my OU degree), I felt that I wasn't getting anywhere. With hindsight, I can see that my plate was over-full, but I still felt as if I was running on the spot.

I decided to go to Belize to reconnect with a family member, and this turned out to be such an empowering experience, almost a journey of self-discovery. For the first time I was able to spend three weeks travelling on my own and met loads of cool people. It was my first proper experience of a Black country. I remember being at the airport and being asked, 'Who are you coming to visit?' As if I just naturally belonged there.

They have every single colour of the rainbow in Belize and speak Spanish and English. For the first time, I felt that I wasn't leading with my race. Without the cultural emphasis on skin colour, you just feel like you're free to exist. I loved it there. I went to the Cayes (tiny islets) and drove around an island on a golf cart, and I visited the ATM (Actun Tunichil Muknal) Cave. The countryside was beautiful, the food was lovely and there was a Caribbean vibe that made me feel at home.

In terms of my own strength of character, that trip was a really big deal. For the first time, I travelled alone and took responsibility for myself. Even though I was scared at first, I pushed through and in the end, I had a wonderful time. Looking back, that trip marked a turning point for me, even though I wouldn't recognise it for a few years yet.

COURAGE

In August 2016, I was leading a settled life: I was working for the civil service, living in the same flat I still live in now in Greater Manchester, and studying and volunteering part time. I didn't know when I woke up on a summer Sunday that an incident that morning was going to change my life for ever. Now I know through bitter experience that, sometimes, everything can change in a second, and a single event can have far-reaching consequences on the way the rest of your existence unfolds.

I had a medical appointment that morning, which was walking distance away. Crossing a main road on the way there, I was standing on a pedestrian island surrounded by railings, waiting for the lights to change. I remember seeing a blue car speed past and thinking to myself, *Oh my goodness!* He was travelling so quickly along quite a slow road, strewn with bollards marking road works that were going on all around.

Then I remember turning 90 degrees to my left and seeing the bonnet of a black Audi coming straight for me. It was travelling so fast, and it was terrifying. In the next second, he had smashed into the barrier and a traffic light inches away from

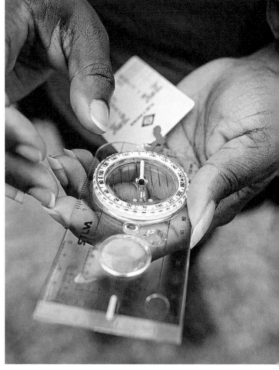

➡ A simple compass is all you need to find your way. © Emily Ward Photography

where I stood. The car was a total wreck. Completely crumpled. But somehow, standing in the middle of the devastation, I was alive, saved by the railings and the traffic light.

It must have been very dramatic for everyone witnessing it. All the traffic stopped and lots of people jumped out of their cars. One man said to me, 'I thought I was going to see you killed then.' Another witness had a dashcam and promised to send me the footage.

A woman stopped her car and asked where I needed to go. She offered me a lift, and I accepted gratefully. So there I was, sitting in her car with her and her mum, when I suddenly exclaimed, 'I think I need a cuddle!' and burst into tears.

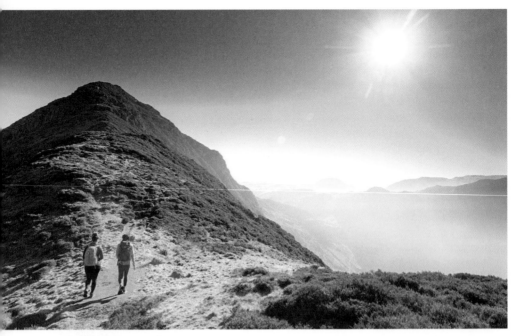

➡ ABOVE: Hiking up Fleetwith Pike.
© Tom Bailey
➡ RIGHT: Ziplining through the gorgeous landscape of Mexico.

People had been really kind but it was all so overwhelming.

When I was sent the dashcam video, I forwarded it on to my family and the policeman who'd turned up at the scene. He told me what I knew: if that barrier hadn't been there, I would have died. I was very lucky that the police pursued it, and I have a full picture of what happened that day. They studied CCTV footage of the crash, which showed the cars racing through the local streets just before the collision.

In the end, the driver was charged with dangerous driving and pleaded guilty. He was only 26. He was disqualified from driving for 12 months, given an eight-month suspended prison sentence for 24 months, and ordered to carry out 200 hours of unpaid work and to take an extended driving test before he could get his licence back. He was also fined £140. I was pleased the driver avoided prison – he was just young and reckless and if he'd hit me, I wouldn't have wanted my death or serious injury to ruin his whole life. Hopefully, he's learned his lesson.

In the weeks and months after the crash I became really anxious. The road where it had happened was very near my home. I had to cross it to get to work every day and every time I felt frightened. I went to the doctor to talk about it and showed him the crash footage. He diagnosed me with PTSD and tried to put me on beta blockers but after chatting with the pharmacist I decided I didn't want to take pharmaceuticals to control my heart rate. It didn't seem like a healthy way to live and I felt like I'd be able to manage it myself.

After a while, I began to understand that this was anxiety, and some of the fear turned to anger. It didn't feel fair that the impact of this near-death experience had reduced me. I didn't feel like I was the strong person I had been before. This whole process took a couple of years – it wasn't instantaneous – and the anxiety created by the accident coincided with other feelings of drift in my career, which compounded its effects. I realised that I needed to do something to get myself out of the rut I was stuck in and this would take courage.

A couple of years after the accident, in the middle of winter, I had been on a week-long course to become an advanced union representative, an extra responsibility to my civil service job. I was travelling back home by train on a beautiful section of the Hope Valley Line that runs through the Peak District – it really is a stunning route, and it's no surprise that it's popular with walkers. Gazing out of the window, I thought about making a New Year's resolution. I wanted to do something productive with my time, but I also wanted to do something that fed my soul: a sense of being part of something; moving forwards and not staying still; enjoying the world outside rather than feeling afraid of it... As I watched all these walkers get on and off the train at different points, I suddenly realised that the answer was right there: I was going to take up hiking. I took a video through the train window and put an update on my Insta status: 'I'm taking up hiking this year' #BlackGirlsHike. Then a few days later I set up my Instagram page for Black Girls Hike.

My volunteering experience showed me that if I wanted to do something, someone else probably felt the same. So, I put out a message asking anyone if they fancied going for a hike. And that's where it all started: me sitting on a train wanting to do something for my well-being and finding the courage to do it. I am still on that journey now.

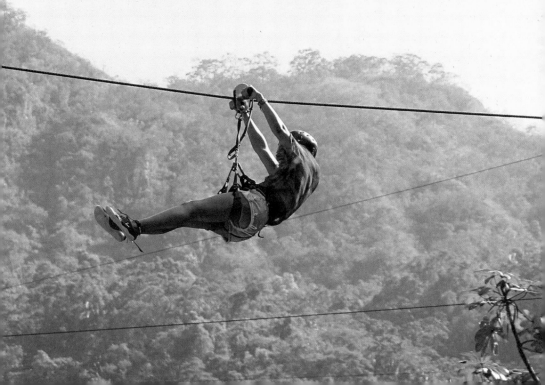

DETERMINATION

I think that for most of us, until you find your path to whatever gives you joy, there are a lot of internal struggles to overcome. I felt I had to do what society wanted me to do, but working all week in an office with my older colleagues who felt to me like a bunch of dragons was like being in prison! But if I had asked myself what I was being trapped by, I wouldn't have been able to answer. It takes a long time to unpack all of this, but at the heart of it is societal expectations.

For young people now things can be harder in some ways than they were for their parents' generation. There are so many factors at work: high house prices, the lack of financial support from the state in areas like higher and further education, as well as the effects of social media. We are able to compare our lives not just with people we know and whose faults we're probably familiar with, but also with the whole seemingly perfect world! As a result, making decisions on how to move forwards in our lives can become more difficult.

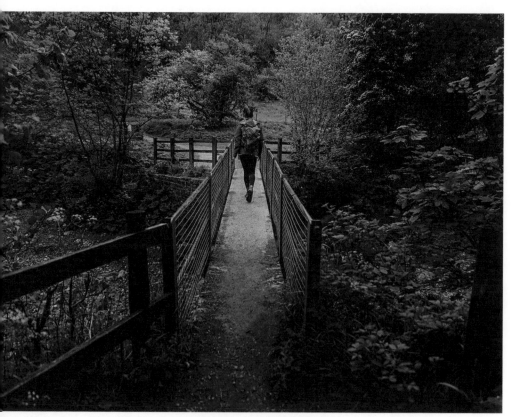

➡ A path near Thor's Cave in the Staffordshire Peak District.

COLLECTIVE WISDOM

Apart from raising public consciousness about the barriers that stand in the way of so many people enjoying the freedom to roam, one of the most important things BGH has given me personally is the chance to meet many women. With countless different perspectives to share, at the end of each walk I have felt myself grow a little. I've had deep and meaningful chats with people I hardly know! It's such a gift to be able to hear wisdom from older women who have been there before. I have got some really great advice, and a sense of ease from these encounters.

For Black women, on top of all of the above, there's the issue that hilling isn't something that our community had traditionally been included in. This is why I created my own group. Because I didn't want to pay $7.99 for the Meetup app, I created an Instagram page that simply invited other Black women who wanted to meet like-minded people to come for a walk around Hollingworth Lake in Rochdale.

This was in March 2019, and at the time I didn't drive so I wasn't able to go and practise the hike before I did it. In the end, I was an hour late turning up because I had to wait for a lift from my sister! When I eventually arrived, I was amazed to find 14 women waiting for me. Though at this stage I hadn't had any training, I led the hike, and I did go off the route a bit, but I successfully managed to get us back to the start. It was such a rewarding experience. As well as being surprised by how many women had turned up, I found it so wonderful just to be out in the fresh air, meeting new people and talking away to each other like old friends. It was a drizzly day in March, but just by being with these women and doing something new together I felt like we had already created a little community.

I continued to post walks on my Instagram page and the numbers of participants continued to grow over the year. Other Black community groups sent members, and women travelled from all over the country to join us, which showed that there was a pent-up demand nationally for what we were doing. By 2020, we had groups around the country. In August 2020, more than 100 people attended our first London walk around Epping Forest.

As well as giving me a way to overcome my anxiety, leading walks really boosted my confidence. I began to realise that access to the outdoors and green spaces had been what was missing from my everyday life, working nine to five in an office. And it was quickly clear that BGH was providing a safe space for increasing numbers of Black women to explore and reconnect with nature. But it was almost by accident that I ended up founding an organisation which challenged the lack of representation in the rural environment. I didn't set out to be an activist: that came with the whiteness of the territory we, as Black women, were exploring.

It was a friend I'd met through BGH who helped me to make the decision to leave my full-time job. I was still with the civil service, in a stable and secure role that gave me enough time to run BGH alongside it, but only to a certain level. Through her support and encouragement, my friend gave me the confidence to do what was needed to give BGH the chance to fulfil its potential with my full-time attention. This wasn't an easy choice, and it was only when I took that step that I realised how determined I was to bring the benefits of BGH to as many people as possible. At this point, I didn't understand that it would take over my life or that I would become a figure known in the media as a result. I was just giving BGH as much time and attention as it needed. I found that it would take all of it of course, and that it still wouldn't be enough!

> " AS WELL AS GIVING ME A WAY TO OVERCOME MY ANXIETY, LEADING WALKS REALLY BOOSTED MY CONFIDENCE. "

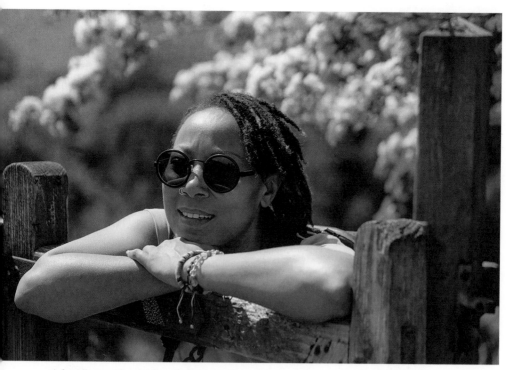

➡ A well-earned rest (above) after kayaking on Brothers Water (right) in the eastern Lake District.
© Photo by Laurelle

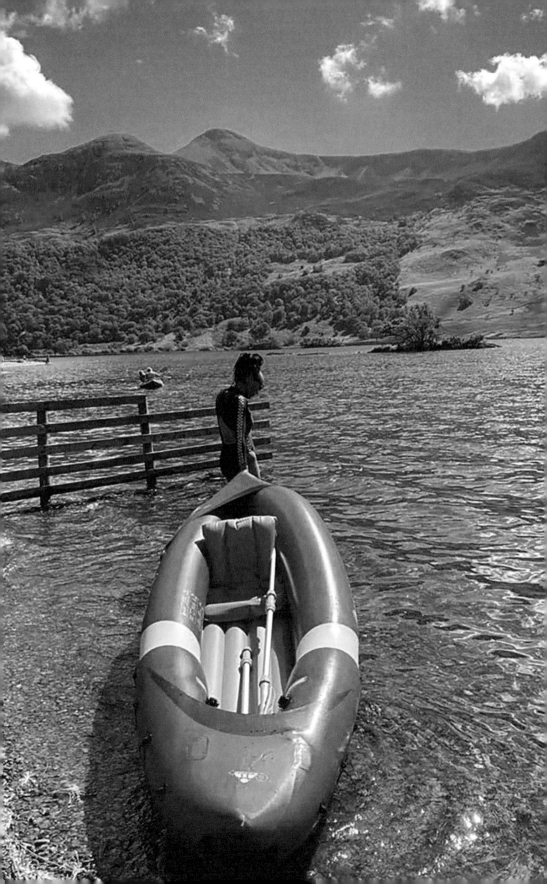

INSPIRATION

Name:

LIZ DRYSDALE

Age:

68

Profession:

RETIRED FORMER BICYCLE INSTRUCTOR

Lives:

WIGAN

I've always loved the outdoors, especially camping and camper vans. And I've always walked – not great distances, but I loved being out in the fresh air. I grew up in Liverpool, and I think I got my interest in the outdoors from gardening and my dad. There were seven of us kids, and my Jamaican dad used to walk with us to Sefton Park, a good few miles away. There was a big glass palm house there, which my dad liked going in because it was warm and they had massive tropical plants, yucca and banana trees.

Then around 15 years ago, I became a cycle instructor and started working for Bikeability, which meant I was outside all the time. After that, I decided that I couldn't work indoors again.

I've never lacked confidence to try new things. I'm a former community activist and was the first Black female councillor in Liverpool in 1987, after the riots. Near the end of my working life, I was putting HGV and lorry drivers on bikes to train them about what it was like be a cyclist on the road. I've always had wild and wonderful jobs – as a youth worker, a community group leader – I've never had a 'career' as such.

When I met my partner, I discovered that he was a keen walker, and we used to go together. Sadly, he passed away in January 2021. While he was alive, we would go walking with a local group in Wigan, who were mostly

white, but I didn't want to walk with them once my partner had died. They weren't friendly enough and frankly, after losing him, I felt quite vulnerable.

This is how I became involved in Black Girls Hike. I knew that after my partner's passing, and even though I was alone, I still wanted to get out. But I wanted to carry on hiking in a safe space where I didn't have to worry about people's attitudes. In other groups I tried I almost had to put my armour on before I went out. I just wanted a space where I didn't have to do that. Where I could relax.

First, I joined a walking club, but people would make race- or class-based comments that would drive me up the wall. When there were fires on the moors, it would be: 'Oh it's *those people*, they're coming out here

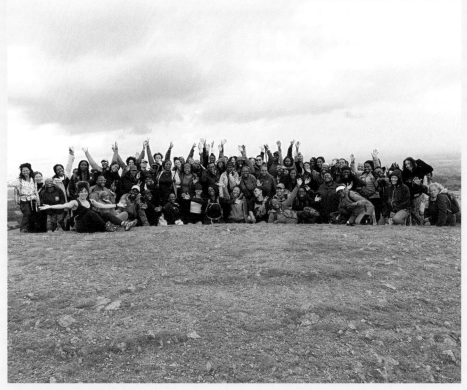

➡ Black Girls Hike is a welcoming community. © Photo by Laurelle

and setting the ground on fire.' And I would be fuming, because there was no evidence for this. It was just a prejudiced assumption. I just didn't feel comfortable spending time with those people.

There is still a lot of work to do in outdoors education to make it a place in which people of colour can feel comfortable. I recently attended an outdoor skills course where I was the only Black woman among the participants. Only in retrospect did I suss out that the main leader of the group would try to undermine me when I had something to say. I am chatty, but I wasn't disrupting the group, I was making relevant comments. For example, it had been raining and I said, 'I'm just going to look in this puddle, to see if there are any tadpoles.' She jumped in with, 'There aren't going to be any tadpoles, it's the wrong time of year.' So I went to look at the puddle anyway and found there were loads!

There were also a couple of other times when she assumed I didn't know anything about the countryside. And, on the final day, she was describing a book about safety on mountains and commented, 'The book has been reprinted, and they've got non-whites in it now.' Why did she have to say that? I felt she was having a pop at me, but perhaps she also sees groups like BGH as a threat. So, in response, I said, 'I object to that. I'm not "non-white", I'm positively Black.' After the meeting was over, one of the other women came over to me, and said, 'I agree with you.' *So*, I thought, *why not say this in front of everyone else?* There I was thinking *I* should leave, that I was in an entirely hostile environment.

I have written to complain to the organisation who put on the course,

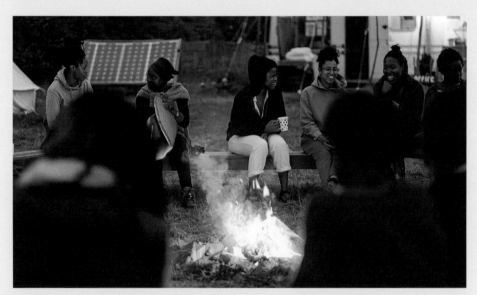

⟹ BGH women chat around the campfire on a camping weekender. © Photo by Laurelle

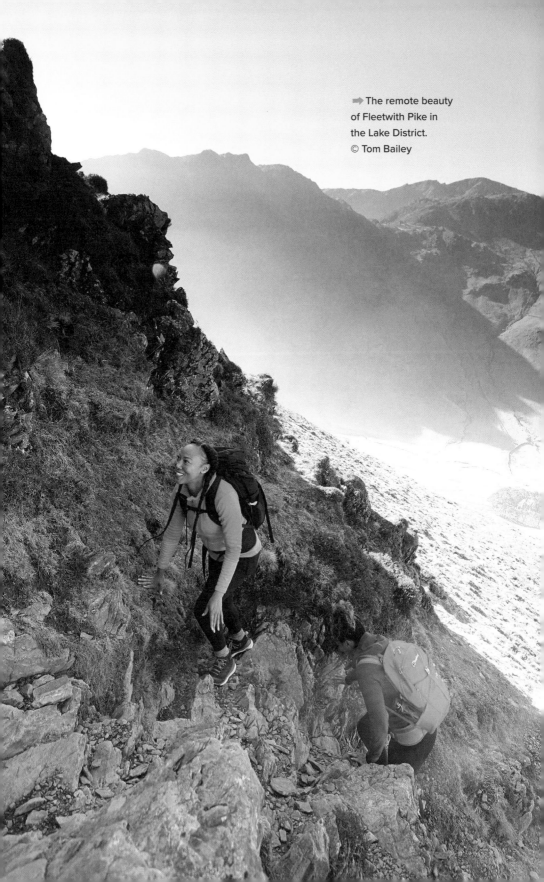

➡ The remote beauty of Fleetwith Pike in the Lake District.
© Tom Bailey

and they wrote back to me saying, 'I'm sorry you were affected by this.' Well, it wasn't just me! Everyone there was affected. This is what I mean: we are treated like exceptions, rather than ordinary people. As I told the instructor, 'I'm 68 and I'm f*****g sick of this.'

What's clear to me is that people like them are making the outdoors an alien place for Black people. In particular, there's an assumption that as Black people we never go into the countryside, and we don't know anything when we get there. When you gain a little knowledge, it gets worse, as you become a potential threat to them. They think you might want to do what they're doing, and they can become quite obstructive. My experience at the course was a good example: I've not heard anyone say 'non-white' in years.

Since my partner passed away, I have bought a tiny camper van, and luckily, I don't mind my own company. I sometimes go a couple of days early to a BGH walk venue, and the walk is something to look forward to. Usually, you'll have a good laugh and people are very supportive of each other. Obviously, you have to adjust to being alone after a partner dies, but if I didn't get to walk then that would be another factor that would simply add to my grief. It would be another loss. It's really important that I keep going.

But, though I enjoy getting out into the countryside, I think that the obstacles that come with it might stop some people like me going. Since my partner passed away I've booked on to a lot of things that are not run by BGH, partly because I'm trying to keep busy, but every time there's been a disaster and I've not gone back. I've thought, *No, I'm not paying money to feel uncomfortable because of their racism*. Sadly, this means that there's another chunk of world I can't get a grip on.

I think Rhiane, and BGH, has opened up this conversation. I admire Rhiane for taking on that challenge. When I was a cycling instructor, I think there were only six Black people doing the job in the whole of the UK, and I knew three of them. There need to be more Black instructors in every area of the outdoors, so that the children see people who look like them. Anyone who takes on that challenge deserves our support.

66
AT 68, I DON'T HAVE TIME
FOR NONSENSE.
99

BELONGING

A big part of what we do at BGH is to make the outdoors more accessible to people who don't feel welcome in rural areas. The work of BGH now influences policy and we collaborate with other organisations to create projects and services, and to increase the opportunities for all people of colour to learn about and experience the natural environment. Though BGH has expanded its areas of expertise, and we now strive to enable opportunities for other people of colour, we still keep our walks, weekenders and holidays focused on Black women. Our more than 5,000 members have found a sense of belonging in BGH and we don't want to let them down.

We've come a long way from my first Instagram page! We're now Black Girls Hike Community Interest Company, and in addition to me there are five other employees and a Board of Trustees who guide the organisation's development.

The biggest surprise to me is how BGH has exposed how inhospitable the outdoors can be to people who aren't white. We talk a lot about Black people facing 'barriers' to enjoying the outdoors.

In fact a lot of these are the same barriers everybody faces: access, time, resources and safe spaces. In addition, minorities do tend to be centred in more urban areas, so as we grow up, we're not as likely to be exposed to the natural environment.

But, more damagingly, a lot of people see the outdoors as a white domain, a space where there is, unfortunately, always the threat of racism and prejudice. The 'outdoors' in this context means more rural areas. When Black people go to rural areas they stand out and it can feel unwelcoming and isolating. Sometimes there's even a hostile reception and we sadly get the message that we simply don't belong.

Sometimes these attitudes are reflected in my experiences representing BGH. I once attended a popular outdoors event where we were called a 'bobsleigh team' – obviously referencing the film *Cool Runnings*. This is a typical example of a microaggression or casual racism, passed off as a joke. I noticed a lot of tokenism. It's easy to get the impression that we are interchangeable, and it's the prospect of these types of

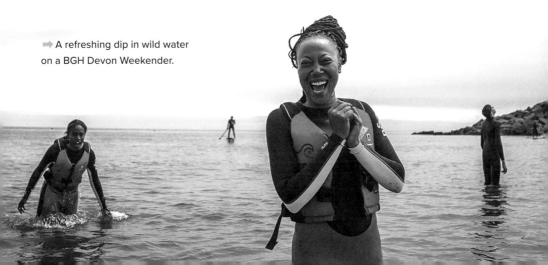

➡️ A refreshing dip in wild water on a BGH Devon Weekender.

GREEN SPACES

When I was in Jamaica in 2018, everything was so green. Going there made me realise how much we're naturally connected to the land and how the ties we have, have been severed over time due to systemic inequalities and all the ways they manifest. Going to Jamaica just reaffirmed that we are from nature and how important it is for us to be immersed in it and feel connected to it.

experiences that puts people off. There's just so little representation. Once, a big group of us was out in the Peak District, walking up a hill. We passed a Black guy walking down, and he had obviously never seen so many Black people hiking before – you could tell by the look on his face, which was priceless. Another time, we were walking through Epping Forest and passers-by kept stopping and asking if we were going to a BLM protest!

The lack of representation travels all

➡ ABOVE: Swimming at Lake Windermere in the Lakes. © Photo by Laurelle
➡ RIGHT: Preparing a hearty meal at a camping weekender near Worcester. © Photo by Laurelle

the way through the outdoors community. We recently held a weekender at which the women did all kinds of outdoor activities, and some of the feedback from our members was asking why we didn't have Black instructors. The simple response was that you just don't get Black instructors in the outdoors, but we knew this wasn't enough of an answer and that we had to do something about it. We originally started working with Mountain Training to train our leaders, but in 2022 we became an approved provider with them, so that we can now deliver those training courses ourselves – the first Black organisation to become an approved provider since Mountain Training was established in 1964. To date, there have only been a handful of women who identify as Black who are qualified as mountain leaders. (You can read interviews with some of the BGH members who have done this later on in the book.)

Through BGH, we want to make the outdoors more aspirational for Black people – so it is something we consider when thinking about where to live and our careers, as well as what hobbies and activities to pursue in our spare time. Sometimes we can combine both, and there are interviews later on with adventurous people who have managed to do just that, living and working in the

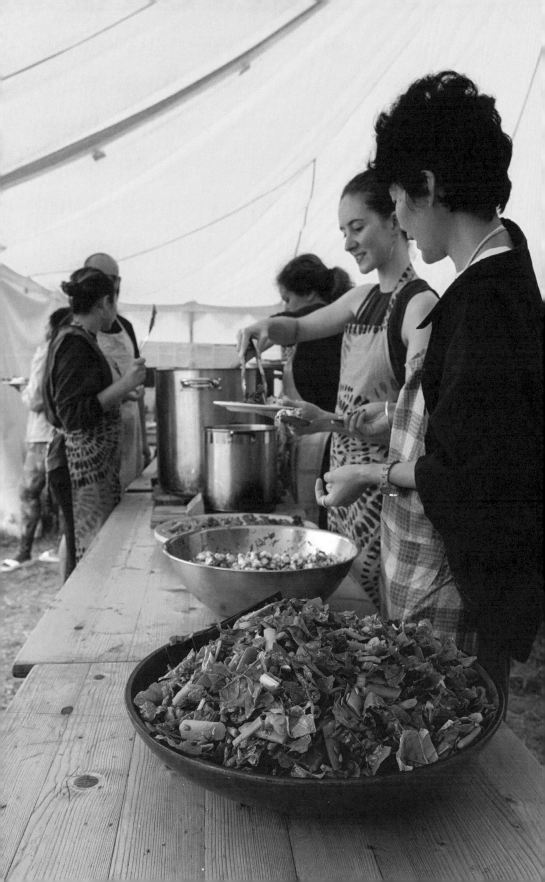

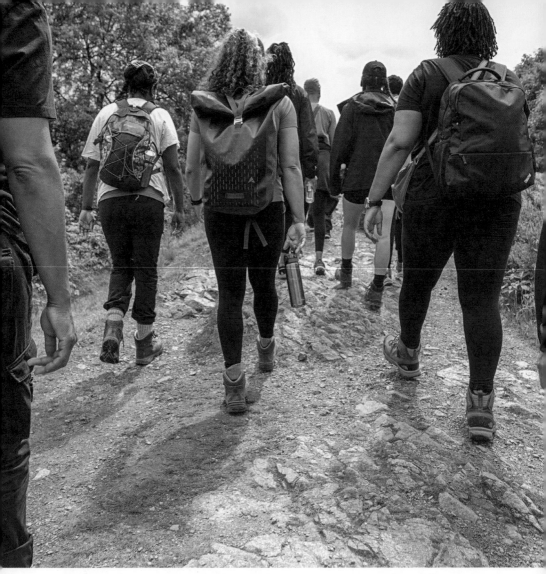

➡ Every journey starts with a single step and starting out is easier than you think. © Photo by Laurelle

outdoors which is a real win-win situation. Over the past year or so, BGH has started to run trips abroad to Madeira, Morocco and Ghana. Ghana especially was so interesting. It was a beautiful, culturally immersive experience and amazing to be back there as a diasporic sisterhood. We all share a real sense of belonging when travelling as a group.

"... WE WANT TO MAKE THE OUTDOORS MORE ASPIRATIONAL FOR BLACK PEOPLE"

COMMUNITY

The community aspect of BGH is so important. By showing up as a group we create a safe space for ourselves and our members to encounter nature, to learn and to grow. It is so necessary, though when I try to explain why, I often encounter resistance. It comes as a shock for people to hear that people of colour are half as likely as white Britons to spend time in nature. When people think of hiking they might imagine a group like The Ramblers, typified by older, white people. (I used to call them 'The Beige Pants Brigade' but someone emailed me to complain!)

Traditional walking groups aren't very attractive to Black women as we are never sure if we are going to stand out, or even how welcome we will be. The truth is, many of us spend our days in jobs where we code-switch to fit into a majority-white environment so, when it comes to our leisure time, we don't want this extra layer of labour – we just want to relax and *not* feel like we have to justify our presence. This feeling is compounded by the lack of diversity of the population in rural areas, and a sometimes unspoken and uninterrogated assumption on the part of people of colour that the countryside doesn't 'belong to them'. So BGH is a vital alternative space for Black women who want to hike, a welcoming community where we don't have to work to 'fit in'.

> ## " BGH IS A VITAL ALTERNATIVE SPACE FOR BLACK WOMEN WHO WANT TO HIKE, A WELCOMING COMMUNITY WHERE WE DON'T HAVE TO WORK TO 'FIT IN'. "

BGH has become a mutually supportive community of women with our common interests in the outdoors at its heart. For example, during the Covid-19 lockdown when restrictions only allowed you to exercise with one person outside your own household, our Facebook group became a place where members could go online to find a local buddy. One of the members created a Google document that allowed members to find a walking buddy close to their location – she didn't have to do that but, as well as exercise, this provided a lot of mental health support for people who may not have had any company at all. When groups of 30 were allowed, we were able to start back up again quickly, running a lot of hikes. It was amazing the way the community sustained itself through the crisis and looked after its members.

One of the most amazing things is that the community works on every level – from novices for whom the outdoors is

COMMUNITY AT THE CORE

Community is important to me. I have been involved in community-building all my working life, and BGH is a natural extension of this. As well as studying community-based organisation as part of my Open University degree, much of the volunteering and studying I did before I started BGH was with various community groups in the North West.

Volunteering was a way to build community around myself when I first moved to my area of Greater Manchester. I volunteered for Refugee Action as an ESOL (English for Speakers of Other Languages) teacher and did advocacy work, such as taking people to register at the doctors or the library. I also volunteered at the ESOL drop-in session, helping with accommodation or with accessing services. I worked with Mothers Against Violence in Manchester, assisting with events, and at a Sudanese charity that raised awareness of female genital mutilation (FGM), for whom I also taught ESOL and ran homework sessions. And of course, being a union representative was also an extension of these activities, as I worked to protect and further the rights of my civil service colleagues.

My volunteering taught me so much about people and what they need from a group; how to make them feel welcome, connected and invested.

completely new, to more experienced participants who were isolated from other Black women. Everyone can find a home at BGH without feeling that they are holding anyone back or don't have the right skills or body shape to take part. BGH members help each other. It's been incredible to see how exposure to the outdoors builds people's confidence and improves their mental health. Helping to make that happen has been so rewarding.

I recently did a trip to Norway to learn kayaking and it was so different to how we run BGH events. There was an undertow of competitiveness between group members and an unwillingness to open up to each other during the evenings when we had little else to do but share our stories. BGH members are so generous and open like that: they enjoy sharing wisdom and expertise, not only about their practical skills, but also about their lives more generally. The awkwardness I experienced on this trip was not something I was used to!

66
EXPOSURE TO THE OUTDOORS BUILDS PEOPLE'S CONFIDENCE AND IMPROVES THEIR MENTAL HEALTH
99

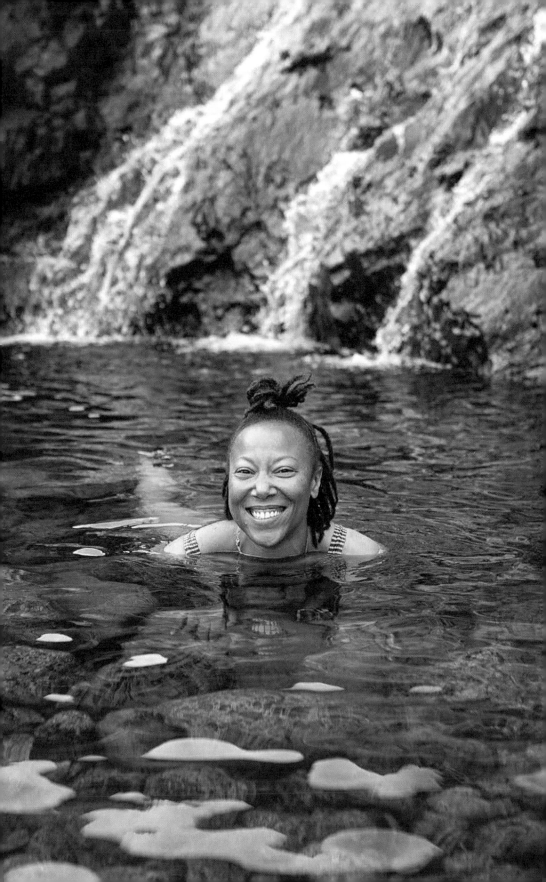

INSPIRATION

Name:

BUSHRA SCHUITEMAKER

Age:

29

Profession:

ZOOLOGIST/PHD RESEARCHER ON POULTRY WELFARE AND AGRICULTURAL SUSTAINABILITY

Lives:

NORFOLK

Photos © Bushra Schuitemaker

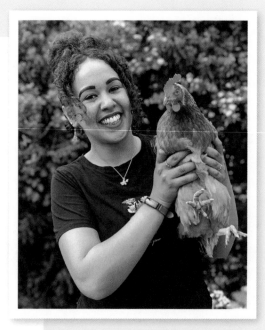

Getting involved with BGH has meant the world to me because it is for people like me. And when we meet up, we're not going into the outdoors to be activists, we are going for a hike. Even though we are creating so much change, it doesn't have the same burden of responsibility. I can be with other Black women and not have to code-switch. We can all relax.

I've always been very outdoorsy — I grew up in rural Essex and enjoyed what I think of as 'countryside privilege'. It was all around me, and I have been obsessed with animals since I was seven years old. I've always loved exploring nature, and especially observing animals in their natural habitat, hence my career path. I kayak and canoe and am into scuba diving. At school, I did my Duke of Edinburgh's (DofE) Awards and was in the Girl Guides.

I was lucky I had the opportunity to do all this, but whether in school or taking part in other activities, I was always the only person of colour. This was partly to do with the area in which I grew up. Once I got to Anglia Ruskin University to study zoology I wasn't quite so alone. Saying that, there were still only two other non-white students on the course, and I

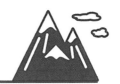

was the only Black British person. In fact, I was often the only woman. And studying life sciences, this hasn't improved. I often do independent surveys to look for eels, otters and water voles, and I am engaged locally in conservation. Even so, I have never felt I had a safe space to be myself and fully experience nature.

I have suffered a lot from imposter syndrome as a result. It's quite isolating when I'm out alone and feel like I am being watched by other people. I've also felt an assumption that people of colour will act inappropriately. I am fully aware of how nature works and when to be quiet around nesting birds, for example. But I think white people are cautious of Black people, more wary of us. Sometimes this surveillance manifests as being overconsiderate when I just want a space to relax.

There have been situations when I might miss out on things. For example, if I come across a bird hide that is busy, I won't go in there. I

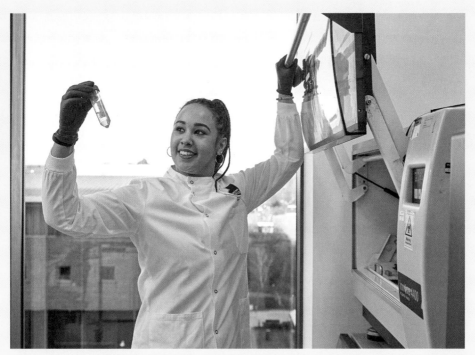

➡ Smashing stereotypes. © Matt Keal

might go for a walk and come back later, hoping that it will be empty when I return. It's that feeling that eyes will be on me, judging me harshly. As a result, I believe that I must demonstrate that I know what I'm doing.

And growing up in a rural white area, I've always been judged by higher standards, and this has led me to put pressure on myself. I feel that I am representing Black women all the time, and that if I do something wrong, people will have the perception that other Black people will do the same. I work with so many committees and work groups to promote racial equality in science and conservation. It can be tiring that the burden of representation falls on the people who suffer most from the lack of it!

For all these reasons, BGH has been really empowering – nature reinvigorates me anyway, but especially so when I experience it with other Black women. Even though we go on really long walks, I have more energy afterwards than when I set out. It makes me happy, reclaiming spaces and sharing in Black joy. We're not hiding ourselves, and I can be out in nature with other people.

❝

IT MAKES ME HAPPY, RECLAIMING SPACES AND SHARING IN BLACK JOY. WE'RE NOT HIDING OURSELVES, AND I CAN BE OUT IN NATURE WITH OTHER PEOPLE.

❞

With my outdoor experience, Rhiane thought I could inspire others, so she asked me to volunteer as a hike leader. I now lead hikes on the Cambridgeshire/Norfolk border. I love being a leader, and I can spot birds, engage with nature and swap fun stories with other women as we go along. This is important to me. With the urgent need to conserve the countryside and its biodiversity, I am doing all I can to inspire a connection with nature in other people.

I've led walks around Ely and Cambridge for between 7 and 15 women. Some are local and some come from London. We start walks from the train station, so that participation isn't dependent on a car. I think this is such a big barrier to accessing the countryside. It is also a major barrier to people finding careers in ecology and the environment. It is unacceptable that a minimum requirement for many jobs is a car and a driving licence. If that is what is required for the role, a vehicle should be provided.

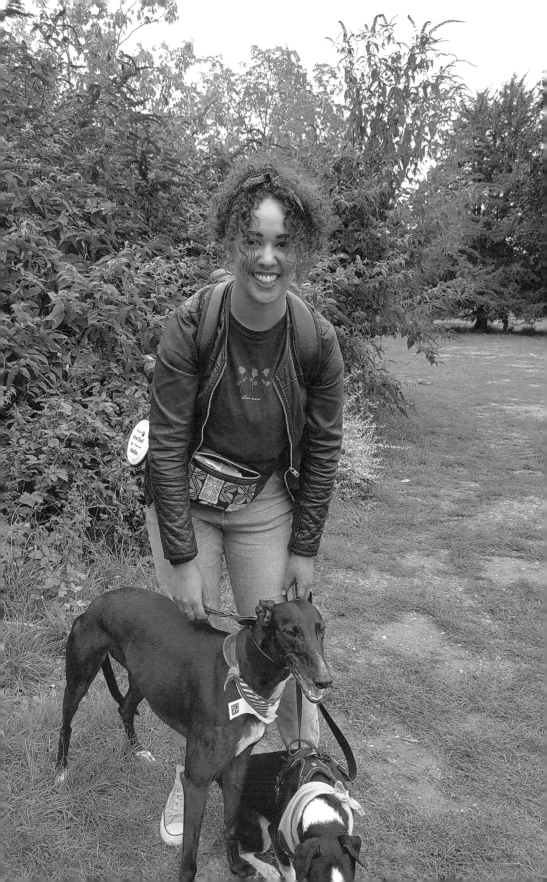

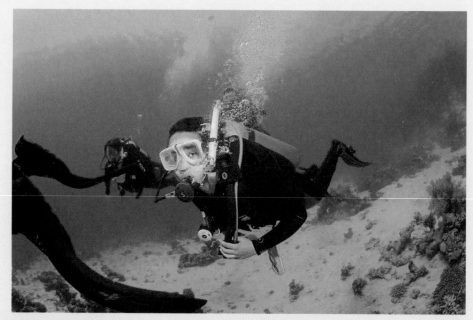
➡ There's so much to explore, on land and underwater.

Historically, there was a safety issue for Black people accessing the countryside. I was more likely to experience strange looks or verbal abuse in rural areas when I was younger, but now I think we have largely moved away from this. I feel much safer in the countryside now – I'm more likely to be patronised than abused. But for generations it has been considered unsafe, and this is the message that people in non-white communities communicate to each other. BGH removes that barrier. Here is a safe space where we can all be together.

There is also a lack of Black history education. Most people don't know that Black people have lived in rural areas for hundreds and hundreds of years. The idea that Black people are only now going into the countryside is ludicrous – we lived in Britain before industrialisation and urbanisation and we sometimes have more of a connection to farming than many white British people who think the countryside belongs to them! There is also an urgent need to diversify agriculture.

Yet the word that the countryside *is* for us is spreading. Recently, my sister joined me on a BGH event, and now she goes to events on her own. She always regarded me and my passion for the natural world as a bit strange – but now she has the bug! I've met so many people through it who have been so amazing and who have learned so much. Recently, for example, I ran a walk in Ely and a woman brought her two teenage daughters along. It was lovely to see them become inspired by the outdoors.

BELIEF

As BGH continued to grow and the effects of Covid-19 lockdowns continued to bite, we came to the attention of the national media, and as the founder of the group, I became the 'face' of the organisation. This has not always been a comfortable role for me. It requires an incredible amount of self-belief. And being increasingly in the public eye has brought with it a lot of pressure. I have had to navigate new spaces and learn to lead an organisation and I have had to invest in my own self-development in order to cope with it all.

When, in January 2021, I appeared on *Countryfile* with journalist Anita Rani to talk about BGH and the lack of access people of colour can have to the countryside, it was the most high-profile piece of media I had done up to that point. The film itself wasn't particularly hard-hitting or controversial, it was just a brown female journalist walking with us and interviewing me and a few of our members about BGH, why I started it and what it means to us. We also talked about some of the issues that work against people of colour coming into the countryside.

In the week before it went out, the producer was in touch offering support because they knew that we were going to attract negative attention. I was so anxious about it I thought, *I just want to be out of the country*. My friend and I went to Mexico on holiday to avoid it, and I didn't even want to be near a TV.

But the reaction to the programme actually being broadcast still came as a shock. Complaints were made to the BBC and we were heavily trolled on social media. It was my first proper onslaught. After it was broadcast, every time I went on the internet, I was just like, *Oh God!* and my heart sank. There was so much abuse. And I did feel personally attacked – I am quite a sensitive person. Setting up BGH was partly about improving my

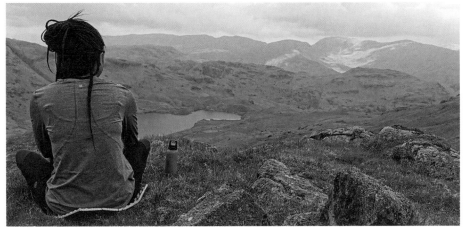

➡ Getting to the top makes it all worthwhile.

mental health, and here they were, so many people who didn't care if they destroyed it. There was someone on Twitter who had over 1 million followers, and another person had commented on his timeline saying, 'Oh they should just hang themselves,' and loads of people had liked it.

The story of the backlash was picked up by other media outlets, including some from abroad. It is a surprise to be open to critique from total strangers. I

once found a thread about myself where one person had put, 'Oh, I've met Rhiane. She's really nice!' but these are not the ones you remember! Learning to have a filter, and proper boundaries, is essential.

It became clear that many people thought that, by drawing attention to the lack of diversity in the countryside, we were somehow stirring up racism. They seem to think that we don't have the same interests as white people, that we lack the ability to lead or build an organisation. This experience also brought home to me how I had gone from being an 'ordinary person' relatively under the radar, to someone with a public profile.

Other groups of people of colour have been on *Countryfile* since then. When the show's own host, Dwayne Fields, addressed the issue by discussing a DEFRA report that found significant amounts of people of colour feel unwelcome in green spaces on the show, it caused another media storm just months later. The *Daily Mail* headline was: 'Countryfile sparks race row' – nonsense of course, as he was only reporting on what DEFRA's own research had found. Twitter again went into meltdown, with calls to defund the BBC.

In fact, after receiving complaints about BGH's appearance, the BBC put out a very supportive statement, saying:

'The feature on the walking group was part of a programme where the overall theme was to encourage people to make more of their connection with the British countryside during the coming year, including trying to get outdoors more to exercise where possible.

'For a variety of reasons, as the presenter explained, it has been the case that

historically some groups have felt less able than others to take part in outdoor activities such as hiking or mountain walking, so any initiative which seeks to redress that balance is to be welcomed.

'The walking group in this programme is one such initiative and is a reminder that not only is the beauty of the British countryside there for everyone to appreciate, but that all are welcome to enjoy it and to safeguard its wildlife, landscape, and traditions for the future.'

The final point here is very important: Black people, like everybody, need to be part of efforts to protect our green spaces. We are part of the population, and it is our taxes that are spent along with everyone else's on government initiatives to support wildlife and the sustainability of the countryside. Winning over people of colour and persuading them of the importance of preserving the natural environment helps everyone.

> ## " BLACK PEOPLE, LIKE EVERYBODY, NEED TO BE PART OF EFFORTS TO PROTECT OUR GREEN SPACES. "

My feeling is that being defensive or denying that there is a problem is very unhelpful. Uncomfortable, but constructive, conversations around race need to happen, to overcome the feelings of many people of colour that the countryside is not for them.

On my hikes, I have almost always been made to feel welcome, and it is disheartening that Black people feel so excluded. But it is likely that the press coverage received by outdoors

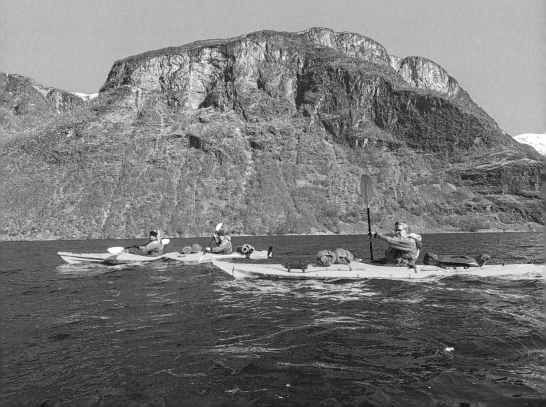

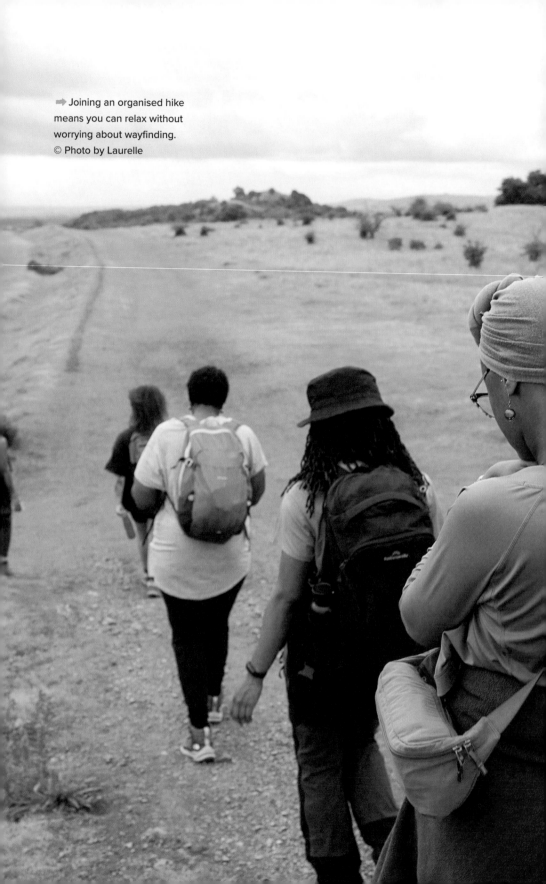

➡ Joining an organised hike means you can relax without worrying about wayfinding.
© Photo by Laurelle

enthusiasts of colour only encourages people to think that the rural environment is not for them.

Reading about the abuse people encounter means it's easy to conflate the trolls who spread hate on social media with the people you actually encounter in rural areas, but they are not the same at all. It becomes a catch-22 – people do not feel comfortable going where they think they won't be welcomed but only by actually getting out there can we counter this.

So, I work hard to promote outdoors adventure but working with the media can be a double-edged sword.

Sometimes, platforms don't do much to support you and quite often comments are not moderated. For example, for International Women's Day, we collaborated with a leading outdoors brand on their Instagram, and their engagement was amazing – much more than they would usually get. But they didn't moderate their comments and it attracted quite a lot of negativity. BGH members often post responses like: 'If you really cared about Black women, you would moderate the comments and not put Rhiane in harm's way.' Which is lovely, but commenting at all only drives more traffic to the problematic content.

LEADERSHIP

It has been a big challenge accepting my role as a leader. I never saw myself this way. After all, when the group first started it was really just a few mates who liked going wandering. Then on one hike, I got us lost on Saddleworth Moor in Oldham. It was a scary moment: the weather was closing in and daylight was starting to fade. I led the group to safety in the end, but it was a real wake-up call. It kind of clicked inside me then: I'm responsible for people, I can't keep getting us lost! After that, I started to educate myself in outdoors skills, including going on a map reading course to give myself more confidence.

That's one of the things I love about BGH – I've had to grow myself to grow the organisation. The first freelance job I had was for City of Trees in Manchester. For a week, I toured the city's parks and decided what the best park was – I couldn't believe I was being paid for it! It

was great, but it was solitary. Now, I have colleagues and partners to train and manage but also many more people I am responsible for. I don't want to let anyone down.

After BGH began to attract attention, I have to admit that, for a while, it did go to my head. I was invited to so many things, and I got caught up in all the whirlwind of new opportunities. But looking back, I stalled BGH's development because it took my attention away from the business element of setting up a Community Interest Company (CIC). I was cherry-picking all the fun stuff and not wanting to do any business admin. Now, my main focus is building a strong foundation for BGH.

Perhaps, on a subconscious level, I suspected that many of the challenges of leadership are rooted in the practical aspects of running a membership organisation, and I wanted to delay it

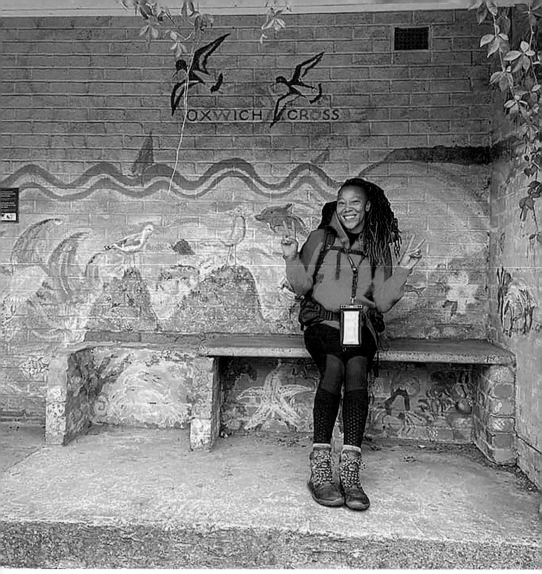

⮕ The multi-coloured bus stop near Oxwich Bay in stunning South Wales.

for as long as possible. This is a joke of course, but seriously, I never realised how difficult it was going to be just meeting all the practical requirements of running events. And, as the group has grown, it's become much harder to organise things. Another challenge was learning how to deal with all the different types of people. It can be difficult to juggle well enough to ensure that everyone is happy.

But learning to deal with difficult personalities is part of the role – you never know who is going to attend an event. Every now and again there will be a challenging personality. But sometimes people are in a very difficult place and this is why they reach out to the group – and I just have to be mindful of that. In those moments, all you can do is try to be professional. Unfortunately, my face tends to give me away as I'm so easy to read. I'm also aware that I can come across as being quite irritable, as I'm often trying to do too many things at once.

However, some of these challenges are rooted in managing a Black-run organisation. People's expectations are very high, and I don't feel like I get a lot of grace from BGH members when we get things wrong. One of our first trips abroad was to Madeira, and we used an external company to run some hikes. On one morning, we thought they were providing breakfast when they weren't. On another trip, the 'hot springs' we had promised turned out to be cold! We spend a lot of time managing people's expectations and we're not perfect, we make mistakes like everyone else.

In terms of working with external organisations, unrealistic expectations can be placed on us because the perception is we're just there to have a good time. There is a commonly held element of resentment that I've heard when serving on boards and panels: 'Oh, I don't like these CICs, they're just people paying themselves to do their hobbies.'

And because we're a Black-led organisation, there's also a higher level of scrutiny. I'm in the public eye and people feel they know me, even though its only via social media and the press, so they expect more of me. They don't have the normal boundaries when they talk to you as you normally would the first time you meet someone. They can be very direct!

But I am told that part of my leadership style is my authenticity. Because I say what I think, candidly and truthfully, people respect that. I come across as very honest, which I am, but this is also the thing that makes me vulnerable to feeling over-sensitive. I am becoming

the leader I need to be, but it's a learning curve.

And as a leader, I have things I want to achieve. I don't want people to put me on a pedestal and be like, 'She's our leader.' I'd like them to be inspired by me and feel empowered that they can do it themselves. Because we're all just normal people. Everybody has that something in them that means they could make a change. It's often just self-belief that women are lacking. So, I don't want them to see me as a leader – I want them to see me as an encourager.

And there are opportunities for advancing the role of people of colour

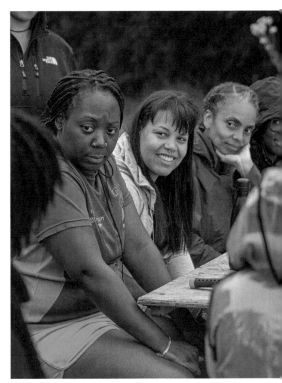

➡ Upskilling women is important so we can take our place in the world of adventure.
© Photo by Laurelle

in the outdoors: now I speak on panels or give talks, and I am listened to. But balancing a public role and running an organisation is difficult – it's easy to give yourself away in small parcels, doing a little bit here and a little bit there, because you are asked, while losing sight of the prize. It's just how society expects Black people to be. Black women have traditionally worked to make other people's lives better and it's ingrained in us.

Now I have stepped into a position of leadership, my network is full of people I used to look up to in the past. That's been great – I can reach out for support to people whom I really respect. Seeing other people believe in me has made me believe in myself. I have always been quite hard on myself, but I am gradually learning to be a bit more forgiving.

There is another layer of expectation that Black professionals have to take on: we have to advocate for our community in unsafe spaces and I've had a lot of hostility from individuals within organisations. Somebody who works for the National Trust, whom I have previously worked with, forwarded my email address to a complainant, so they could email me themselves. There was nothing to this complaint, she was a white person who 'felt attacked' because I had said that the outdoors was not sufficiently inclusive. This is a typical response when people feel challenged because we are discussing inclusivity. There was no need to inform me of this and have me carry that burden. It put me in the firing line and made me feel conflicted. We still have to work with these organisations and this is what we're up against.

This is a kind of insidious racism that is common. Unfortunately, we do occasionally work with people who do nothing to protect us from it. Sometimes I wonder, is it in my mind? Do I have an overactive imagination? Should I be braver?

It has been really, really challenging becoming the leader I've needed to be for BGH. I realised I had a lot of childhood trauma that was being triggered and was coming out in unhelpful ways. To occupy a public-facing role, I had to dig deep and do a lot of healing.

I have had a few experiences in BGH that mean I now feel very conscious of people's intentions when they try to befriend me. You have to learn how to navigate these relationships, because you still need those people to help you grow. It is difficult to work with people sometimes, but it requires me to see the bigger picture and to realise that I'm the leader *for* the BGH community, not just 'of' it. My role serves them, not myself.

" I DON'T WANT THEM TO SEE ME AS A LEADER – I WANT THEM TO SEE ME AS AN ENCOURAGER. "

➡ BGH is a community. © Photo by Laurelle

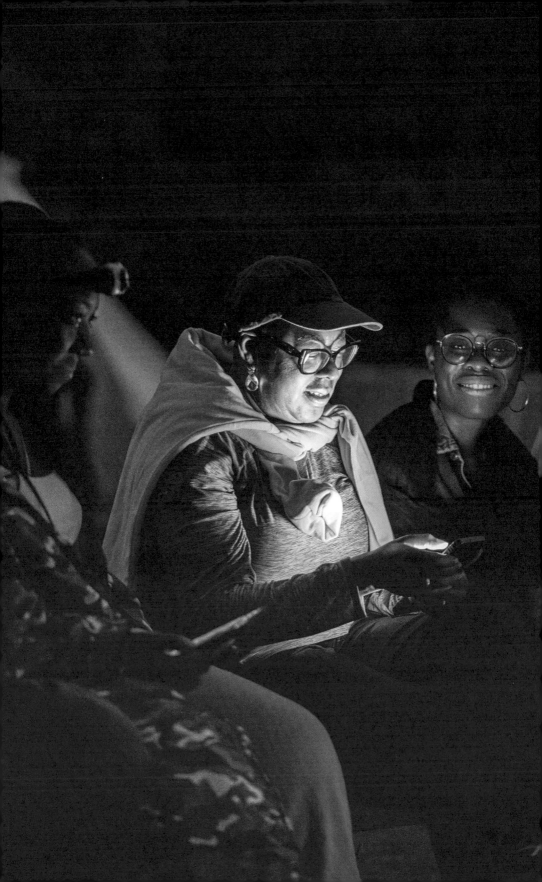

INSPIRATION

Name:

CARLA KHOURI

Age:

48

Profession:

OUTDOOR LEADER

Lives:

ROMFORD, ESSEX

Photos © Carla Khouri

I grew up in Tottenham on a council estate, one of four kids with a single mum. We didn't go on walks or anything like that, but we did have a massive garden and mum loved gardening. She had a manicured lawn and flower borders and we had the rest of the garden, which grew wild. There were stinging nettles, an apple tree and a cherry tree — it felt like a proper wilderness to us kids.

Then when I was a teenager, about 13 or 14, a friend invited me to go with them to the Air Cadets. We were lucky — we had these brilliant ex-military instructors who were very aware of the demographic of the children they were dealing with. We had camps and expeditions, and I did my Duke of Edinburgh's Awards with them — Bronze, Silver and Gold. I left at 18, and my first holiday without adults was backpacking around the Lake District on my own. It was a great experience and from then on, I would go out into green spaces whenever I could.

After university and training as a biology and chemistry teacher, I was really keen to get involved with the Duke of Edinburgh's Award. I led on this in my two secondary teaching jobs and am so proud that I have

helped literally hundreds of young people to enjoy the outdoors. Some of them really took to it and a few took DofE Gold Awards or have done degrees in outdoor education. It's the kind of experience that can change the course of people's lives. During the holidays, we always took my own children camping, making the hikes progressively harder.

In the last few years, I've become qualified as a Summer Mountain Leader. It's a qualification based partly on experience, and before you can get on to the training course you need to have quite good experience in mountainous conditions. For a while, every Friday night I'd get in the car and drive to Snowdonia or the Lakes, to get enough 'mountain days'. Once you have enough, there's a week-long assessment. It's a leadership qualification, so your navigation skills using a paper map and compass must be on point. You also need to show you can work with ropes on steep ground, with suitable kit. It's intense, but rightly so. People need to be assured that leaders' knowledge is sound and we can manage in challenging environments.

You also have to compete hard to get on the course, and there are very few Black women in this area. Since the award was set up in 1960s,

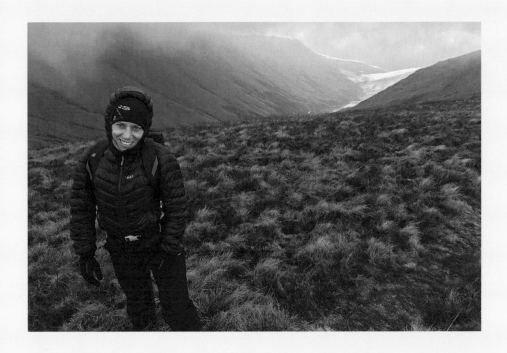

around 25,000 people have qualified, and out of that, only about 4,000 are women. Out of those, the number of Black women who have achieved the Summer Mountain Leader Award is just two!

Now, I have decided to leave teaching and use my qualifications professionally. It was a difficult decision to leave the job I love, but I'm not getting any younger. While I am physically able to, I wanted to give it a go. I'm now working towards the Winter Mountain Leader Award. I really want more Black women to get into the outdoors and leadership roles in the outdoors. This is my way of showing it's possible.

> ## 66
> ## I REALLY WANT MORE BLACK WOMEN TO GET INTO THE OUTDOORS AND LEADERSHIP ROLES IN THE OUTDOORS. THIS IS MY WAY OF SHOWING IT'S POSSIBLE.
> ## 99

I am hoping to work with BGH to train walk leaders, and hopefully give them a flavour of what leadership looks like. I am also looking at passing on my paddle sports and bushcraft instruction skills. I'm qualified as a game ranger in South Africa and can take groups into the wilderness. When I did this qualification I had quite young children – that was a real family adventure!

I've always felt that the outdoors belongs to everybody. I was always aware that there were very few Black families accessing the countryside, but I love the outdoors and I am glad that BGH is showing that the appetite is there. I've never been intimidated, and I don't care that I'm a 5ft 1in (1.55m) Black woman – nothing scares me!

But because so few people like me get experience of the outdoors, they don't necessarily have the idea of working in the outdoors sector. Until you get out there, you won't necessarily know that you want to do a leadership qualification. I think there will be a change: I think there will be more women getting involved. The DofE awards in my schools were taken by lots of female pupils. If anything, at Bronze level there were more girls than boys getting involved.

Getting outdoors is a gift for life, and there are so many physical benefits. I do lots of other sporty things and hiking has enabled me to

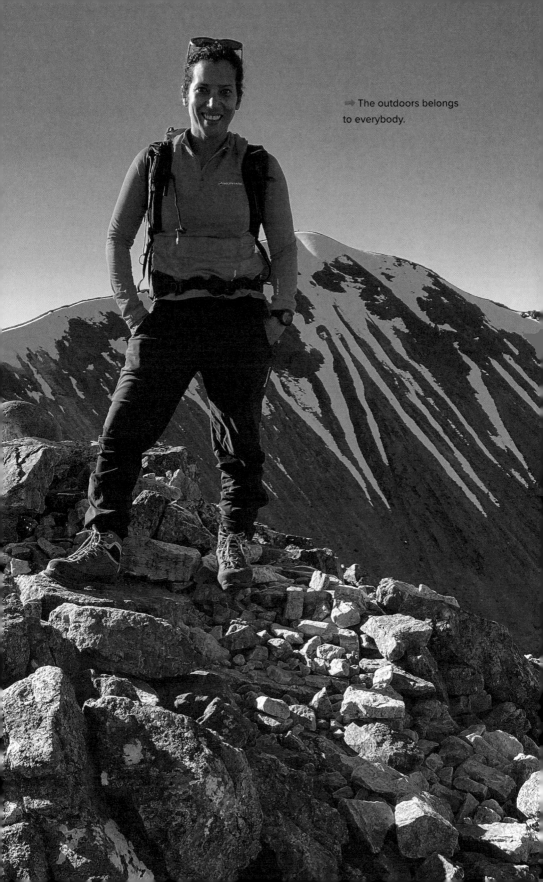

The outdoors belongs to everybody.

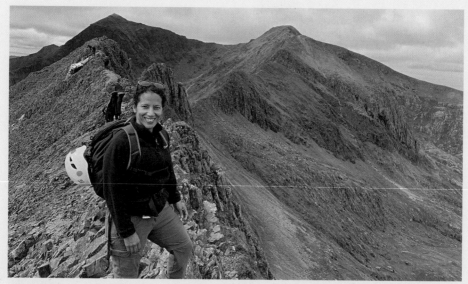

➡ Hiking is an ideal way to maintain life-long physical fitness.

maintain my physical fitness as I've got older. Mentally, if I've been stuck at home all day behind a computer, then getting out into green space is restorative. Throughout my life, and especially when my children were small, heading outdoors was a way of resetting. And socially, it is a real boost. I have made some really good friends through hiking – being outdoors loosens women's tongues, maybe because we don't walk face to face but shoulder to shoulder.

I'm also currently working on a project with Merrell, the outdoor brand, to encourage more women into the outdoors. Interestingly, I have found that being the face of the group means more Black women are joining in. I am keen on inclusivity of generation as well as race and gender. I want women of my age, who have gone through a bit of life and are still active and wanting to share that, to join. I hope that people who come for a hike or a paddle are a little bit inspired to try new things, and to know that you *can do it*. Some women have said they've been scared to try something new, but my story has given them a push to give fresh activities a go.

This has been an adventure for my family, too. My husband and my boys are really proud of me, as is my mum, though she doesn't understand that a woman can be on her own and climb up mountains for fun! She really worries about me, especially now that I'm concentrating on my Winter Mountain Leader qualification. I spent January and February in Scotland in 2023 to get my mountain days in and practise the skills I need. In winter 2023/24, I hope I will have done enough to get on to the training part of the programme. In the right kit, mid-winter is beautiful, magical ... I absolutely love it.

FRIENDSHIP

Friendship is at the heart of BGH and I have made some really strong connections through the organisation. The pandemic made me aware that I was starving for deeper bonds with other people. As a result, some of my pre-BGH friendships haven't stood the test of time because of how much I've evolved as a person.

I have grown out of friendships that were based on going out partying. At first BGH was a fun endeavour, but it has become pretty all-consuming, so I haven't had the time to be as present as I'd have liked to be in my current friendships, or give the time required to strengthen my connections. I would like to make connections more of a priority.

One big difference it that a lot of my friends have settled down and had kids. One of my best friends has had four! She hasn't got time to scratch her arse, never mind have a meaningful conversation. As people's lives inevitably change over time, I miss some of the connections I used to have even if this is just a phase within a friendship rather than the end of anything.

On the other hand, I've met some extraordinary people in the last few years, and have loved working and connecting with them. I aspire to have the same sort of longevity in my field as they've had in theirs, and it's been so empowering learning from this 'girl boss collective'.

I did initially get imposter syndrome when entering certain spaces and feeling awe when meeting high profile individuals, but that doesn't happen now: these are people I can relate to and we're often working in partnership or with shared goals. I wouldn't be in these spaces if I wasn't meant to be there.

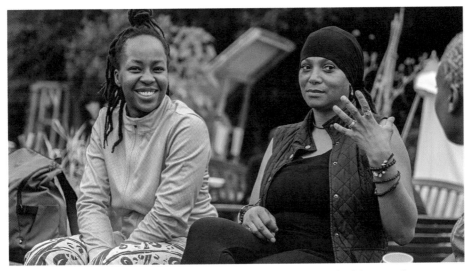

➡ Being in the outdoors strips away everyday barriers to forming meaningful connections.
© Photo by Laurelle

INSPIRATION

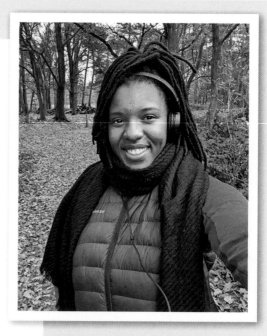

I didn't grow up in an 'outdoorsy' family: that was seen as stuff white people did. I did go on school residentials to Wales, staying in dormitories and going hiking, kayaking and rock climbing, but my real connection with nature came in my early 20s, when I started to become more conscious of my identity.

I joined a reggae band as a singer on my journey of discovering my cultural heritage. In Jamaica, everyday life is centred around nature, through for example walking to school, working outdoors or growing your own food. In the UK, a lot of those connections have become detached. I live in the city, but a lot of reggae music is inspired by nature. Rastafarianism is about getting close to the earth.

I found an allotment around the corner from my house. And at about the same time, I started walking. Only now do I realise I had no clue what I was doing! I would search for a green area, then drive or walk there and just follow the blue dot on Google maps. It doesn't show topographical features, so I had no idea what I was going to encounter.

At the same time, I found it so frustrating that I didn't see more Black people outdoors and spending time in nature. I could see the benefits for me and I wished people from my community could experience them. In 2019, I put an Instagram out about this, and someone replied saying, 'Have you seen BGH?'

I actually remember the feeling of seeing that message. To be honest, I thought I was alone – the only Black woman who liked hiking! A few years ago, representation barely existed, so the appetite for experiencing nature came as a surprise. Social media has been so important, and visualisation is key. If I can't see a picture, I'm going to be cautious; but a photograph of Black women in the outdoors is convincing.

For my first BGH walk, I drove two hours to the Peak District to join in. I hadn't travelled out into these intimidating spaces before but I loved it! I soon became BGH's first Regional Leader. All my walks were in the Midlands, and it was the start of BGH branching out. Since I was responsible for other people, with BGH's support, I learned how to navigate and to read a map on a Mountain Training course.

Now I run a local multicultural walking group for men and women across

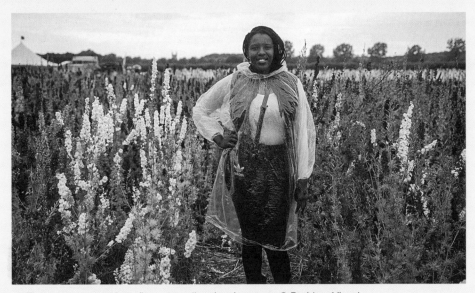

➡ There are so many benefits to spending time in nature. © Brobbey Visuals

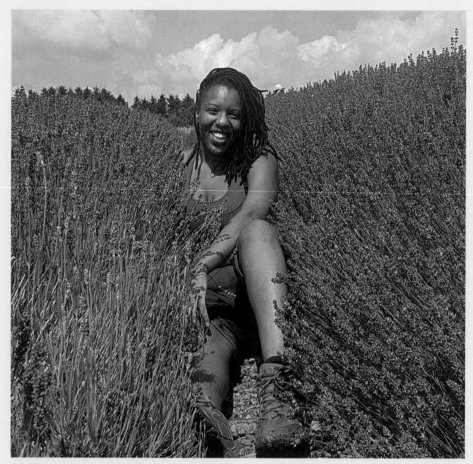

➡ ABOVE: Making a connection with nature.
➡ RIGHT: I try to incorporate outdoor activities where I can. © Brobbey Visuals

the generations called Steppers. I enjoy it and I'm happy to let it become whatever it can be. Some members use it as a workout, others as a chance to connect with other people from the community. I had wanted to do Steppers for years, but BGH showed me how it could work.

It is really about *connection* – this can be completely different for each person. It is a rare space in which people who aren't white can relax and experience a sense of uncomplicated joy at being in nature. It could be hugging a tree or walking around barefoot. But it could just be spending time away from the city, and not hearing traffic. For far too long there have been perceived 'right ways' and 'wrong ways' to enjoy the outdoors. But this is a myth: there isn't a wrong way, provided that you're looking after the environment.

And if someone hasn't been out into the countryside before, they're going to get things wrong. I don't think we should be so heavily critiquing

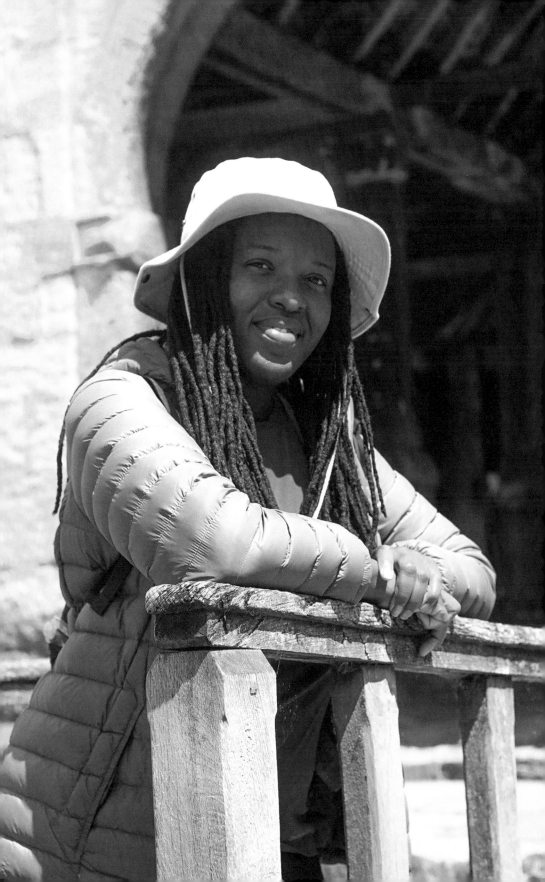

people who make mistakes. For example, when I first started, I might have eaten a piece of fruit and thrown the core into a bush. I used to think that this was OK, but fruit doesn't deteriorate in the same way in the wild as you might expect. And can you imagine the effect on the environment if everyone just threw their food waste around? When this was explained to me, it seemed obvious. Now, I am mindful of the fact that not everyone is experienced and may get things wrong along the way – and that's OK.

This is particularly the case in my work with young people, for which I try to incorporate outdoor activities where I can. Some young people haven't been hiking before and may not do it again for a while. But they may later find that, when they're stressed, they go back to it. Now, or in five years' time – it doesn't matter. I just want to plant that seed.

Connection with my identity, sisterhood and scenery really sum up my experience of BGH. During the Covid-19 pandemic, so many of us needed that connection. BGH supported me, and I am forever grateful to them for training me to lead. And they provided kit to those who don't have it. These days, I am very conscious of the cost of kit and I can give good advice to others, so they don't waste money on the wrong stuff.

I think being put off the outdoors has stopped a lot of people of colour from taking part in these activities – and I have a lot of love and gratitude for BGH for giving me these opportunities. To go into different spaces and lead confidently, knowing I have the right gear and can inspire others, has been a massive confidence booster. But building this confidence does take time. I would be lying if I said I didn't still have feelings of uncertainty when venturing out. I am just lucky that I have the confidence to overcome it.

66

FOR FAR TOO LONG THERE HAVE BEEN PERCEIVED 'RIGHT WAYS' AND 'WRONG WAYS' TO ENJOY THE OUTDOORS. BUT THIS IS A MYTH: THERE ISN'T A WRONG WAY, PROVIDED THAT YOU'RE LOOKING AFTER THE ENVIRONMENT.

99

WELLNESS

The mental and physical health benefits of exercising outdoors are well-documented, and when I started to hike I was aware I needed to do something to enhance my own well-being. Sometimes, things have to get quite bad before you reach outside of yourself and try to change them. Just identifying where you are at can be a massive breakthrough — at least knowing that you're unhappy is a starting point. Getting to the place where you recognise that need in yourself can take time.

Before taking up hiking, I did a course called '5 ways of wellness', which encouraged me to do small things to enhance my everyday life. It was a great starting point, and the suggestions were simple, such as noticing the detail in my environment when I walked and getting

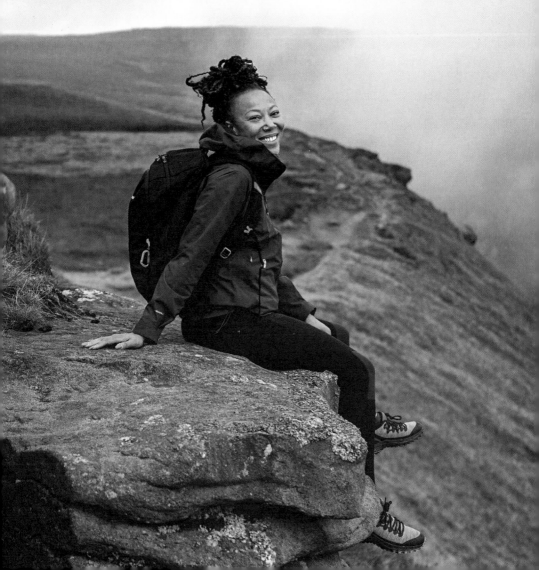

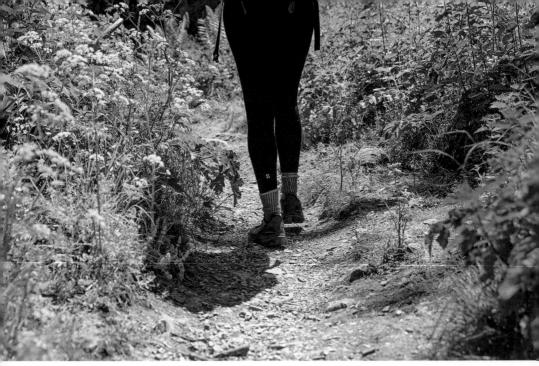

→ Getting into the outdoors was an essential step in improving my peace of mind.
© Photo by Laurelle

a bird feeder (I still love mine, watching all the different kinds of visiting birds). Basically, it was adding things into my life that gave me joy. I learned to appreciate slowing down and paying attention to things outside of my own thought processes.

So, for me, wellness is represented by peace of mind. There are so many elements to this: connectedness, feeling healthy, being emotionally grounded, enjoying strong relationships and having firm personal boundaries so it is difficult for outside forces to disrupt that peace.

Here are some key steps I have taken to boost my peace of mind:

• Learning to do things alone. It's so easy to live our lives seeking permission; first from parents, then partners, then your bosses at work. Living to please other people can mean being afraid to reach out and find your own happiness. I've seen this again and again at BGH,

where women often come alone to events and find a freedom in doing it. So often, BGH has given people a way into an activity that they didn't realise they needed in their lives, but which has brought them great joy.

• Learn to be part of a group. Being in a group where you can connect with people through a shared interest will enhance your growth, offer you different perspectives and prevent you from stagnating in life. When you're hiking with people you barely know in a completely new environment, it's easier to take them at face value. I never ask companions, 'What do you do for work?', but rather, 'Where have you travelled from?' Or, 'What do you do that brings you joy?' By doing this, I avoid playing to my own unconscious biases about professional hierarchies or social class. To keep on challenging your expectations in this way enables growth.

- Travel. It's a cliché but true: travel is a great way to open your mind, encounter new cultures and challenge your long-held assumptions. I have so many stereotypes in my head. Before I spent time in Gambia, I would have scoffed at traditions that appeared to me to be culturally backward. But my attitude is a result of being so Westernised, and not appreciating how rooted these rituals are in history and meaning. I learned that there were lots of aspects of African culture that are traditions that I've not been raised in and haven't fully understood or appreciated. Travelling for me has meant opening up to try to understand these things a lot more.

By taking up hiking and starting BGH, I discovered that these three factors were key to feeling mentally well. And taking my mental health seriously has been a journey in itself. After the near-miss of the car crash, it took me a long time to identify the symptoms of PTSD I suffered as anxiety, not just an aspect of my personality. In all honesty, it was less threatening to think of myself as being a 'worrier' rather than to acknowledge my own biases around mental health. I used to think of mental suffering as a weakness, whereby you are not your full self, but somehow reduced. Now I see managing my mental health as part of life and seek out opportunities for growth and self-development.

From this point of view, BGH was one of the first things I did for my own wellness. Starting and growing the organisation has challenged me in terms of how I manage my emotions. Because I didn't learn how to manage or express my emotions as a child, I feel I am now having to do this in the public eye.

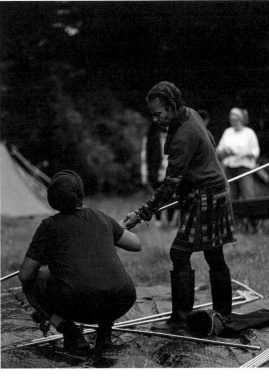

➡ Seeking out opportunities for growth and self-development can boost mental health.
© Photo by Laurelle

> ## 66
> ## I LEARNED TO APPRECIATE SLOWING DOWN AND PAYING ATTENTION TO THINGS OUTSIDE OF MY OWN THOUGHT PROCESSES.
> ## 99

It is part of being an effective leader, but also a well-balanced person, that I want to come across as level-headed to the staff and members. But I also want to *feel* like the best version of myself. Therapy has been part of the journey but I have recently stopped seeing one therapist who I felt was too passive. There was no plan for progress and breakthroughs were few and far between. I think I need to be challenged to bring the best out of myself.

All this work is so necessary. Self-development for me isn't a luxury, it makes what I do possible. Being put into the public eye, leading an organisation, having other people's expectations resting on your shoulders while navigating all these new spaces – it's a lot! I feel I have had to become a bigger person in order to cope with it all.

The attention does make me anxious. Now, I don't know if people are watching me because I look different, I'm well-known or they know me personally. If I meet people who are open in their admiration, I find it very awkward. One woman I met recently was fangirling a bit and asked me to sign something for her. I was so embarrassed at this positive attention that I wanted the ground to swallow me up. Sometimes I feel like I'm giving too much away – my face is very expressive – but then I've never been a surface person anyway!

⇨ The wild flowers of the Peak District. © Photo by Laurelle

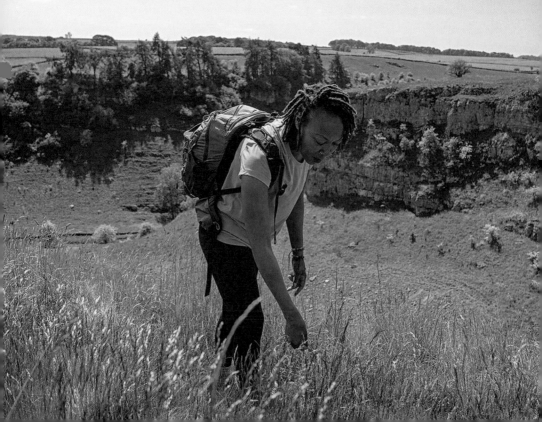

ACHIEVEMENT

I've had many proud moments since I started Black Girls Hike, including taking my mum to Buckingham Palace when I was invited to talk by the Duke of Edinburgh's Award, and earning the recognition of my community when I was named as a Positive Role Model at the 2021 Diversity Awards. Perhaps most memorably, because it was the first time I was invited to a really formal event on behalf of BGH, was when I attended the Women of the Year Awards and surrounded by celebrities and the great and the good from politics.

Awards are all very well, but I feel that the way that we all, as a society, measure achievement is very limiting. Now, in contrast to my twenties, I do feel I am getting somewhere in life, but it's because I am living a life that feeds my soul, not because I am standing on stage giving talks or collecting prizes. It is lovely for all our hard work at Black Girls Hike to be recognised, and all that stuff is really useful for shining a light on the organisation and bringing it to the attention of more people whom we can help and inspire.

I felt very differently just a few years ago. I spent my twenties feeling very anxious about what I *hadn't* achieved. Turning 30, I worried a lot about what milestones I had missed in life, and what that meant for my future. I felt like my friends were overtaking me. I had expected to go to university, enter a graduate training programme, have a good job, meet a partner and have kids. When these things didn't automatically fall into place, I started to fret about where I had gone wrong. What would my future look like? We feel like we've got to meet certain milestones in our lives: university, marriage, kids. There's not much room for any other kind of achievement: creative, non-financial, stuff that's going to fulfil you. I didn't feel like I was achieving anything in life. But I was, I was being proactive about what I wanted to do.

For example, I'd been told my whole life that I had to have a degree to get anywhere. So, by my mid-twenties I had been in higher education twice and

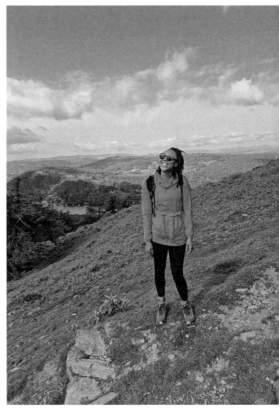

➡ Looking down from Gummer's How.

had started two different courses at two different universities. I didn't last longer than a year at either of them. Looking back, the courses I chose were very academic, which I now know simply wasn't for me.

This can be even more difficult if you come from a family like mine. My father's African culture highly values education. This is also the case on my mother's side: she and her siblings have all got degrees or professional qualifications. Having a degree became a natural part of my expectations for myself.

Don't get me wrong, I love learning (and every day has been a school day since starting BGH!), but I learn best by doing, not by listening and reading. Since I realised this, I've met lots of people who are the same. We can contribute just as much to society as book learners. We are proactive and have great ideas, but we may not have many formal qualifications.

I reached my goals by going the long way around – and that's worked out just fine. Life doesn't have to go from 'A' to 'B' in a straight line. Finding a passion I could develop into a profession took time and luck. But, for all of us, finding that passion means listening to ourselves, and making a positive effort to find out what makes us happy.

To tune into our needs and wants, particularly as Black women, can be difficult. We are often brought up to put other people's needs before our own, which means that making time for self-care and safeguarding our own wellness can be challenging. When I became concerned about how I was using my time, I was very aware of the need to look after myself both emotionally and physically.

Lockdown was a turning point for me and many other people. Small steps helped me to find the joy in things I might have otherwise taken for granted. I consciously look around as I walk, taking time to look up and down and around, taking in every detail. These exercises in concentration and appreciation have really enhanced my everyday journey through life.

Similarly, the BGH achievements I am most proud of are not necessarily the most eye-catching. Last year, the Royal Geographical Society included me and BGH in its awards. We won the Geographical Award for contributions to inclusive and ethical practices in expeditions and fieldwork. This means our efforts to enhance outdoors education has the highest stamp of approval (so we know we are doing something right!).

BGH can now award certificates for young people doing Bronze Duke of Edinburgh's challenges. And we have approval from Mountain Training to train our regional leaders in mountain skills. This sets them up to become the outdoor instructors of the future.

I am so proud of these things because they will form part of BGH's legacy. They are long-lasting – we build professional skills among our members and children so that Black women and their families will become a permanent part of the countryside. This really *is* an achievement – creating something that lasts into the future to inspire future generations.

Even so, I have never worked as hard as I do now! If I could speak to my younger self, I'd tell her she must put the work in. Because short-term discomfort is worth it for the long-term gain of reaching your goals. Choosing discomfort, choosing to do things right, instead of what's easy and comfortable, is what's got me where I am today. But it has to come from an authentic place: you won't prosper in a job that isn't right for you or doesn't suit your temperament.

Ultimately, reaching out into the unknown, as I did, may be the only way to find your path.

"

... FINDING THAT PASSION MEANS LISTENING TO OURSELVES, AND MAKING A POSITIVE EFFORT TO FIND OUT WHAT MAKES US HAPPY.

"

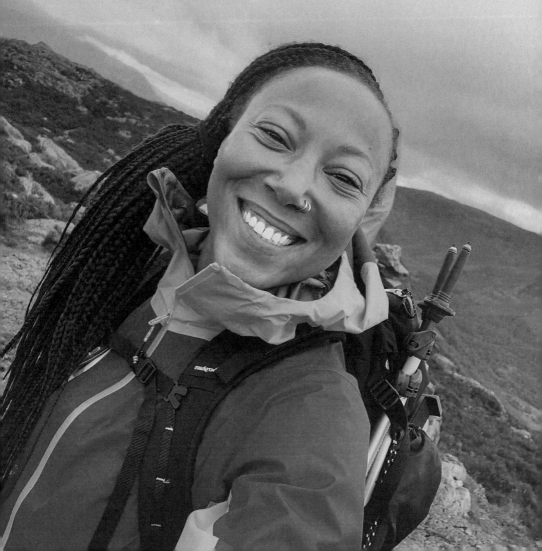

INSPIRATION

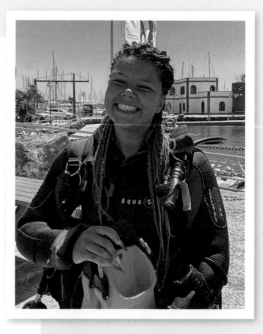

Name:

AMELIA HURSHAM

Age:

24

Profession:

MARINE BIOLOGY GRADUATE

Lives:

TIPTREE, ESSEX

Photos © Amelia Hursham

I've always loved being outside, spending time in nature, and I have always preferred animals over people. I grew up in Witham, which wasn't super-rural. But when I was young, my mum was in poor health and the open spaces around Witham, especially the River Brain, were a real escape. I always knew I wanted to do a job that involved being outdoors. For me, it is as necessary as breathing.

A big part of being in nature is feeling close to my mum. She worked in hair and beauty and was the last person you'd think of in relation to the natural world. She passed away in 2014, but the rape fields coming into flower in spring always remind me of her. It is Mother Earth showing me that there's still love and beauty in the world.

I have a Guyanese/Scottish background and I came across BGH on Twitter. I took the leap when I saw a walk at Seven Sisters in East Sussex. I turned up and sat in the car park for half an hour. It turned out that only I and the leader had come! No one else turned up, so the leader and I did the walk together.

At the time, I had got my degree, but was having trouble finding my place in the conservation/environment sector. This was the first time I'd had an in-depth conversation with someone who had found the sector to be the same as I did. It was so eye-opening to discover that someone else had faced the same barriers as me in getting a job in this field.

My second walk was at Chartwell, and the sense of community was so heart-warming. It genuinely felt healing. It's just so important to be taking up natural space and enjoying it in whatever way feels best for us as individuals. You can play in leaves, sing, dance, have a bit of lunch, whatever. And yes, we can get odd looks, but being present in a group takes the edge off.

It turned out that joining BGH would give my career a real boost, too. In 2021, the Royal Society for the Protection of Birds (RSPB) launched the Greener Thames youth programme. They recruited through diverse organisations – BGH and Muslim Hikers, among others – to attract young people from under-represented backgrounds who wanted to build a career in conservation.

Coming from a science background, I'm very passionate about the fact that we need everyone to be involved in tackling the climate and

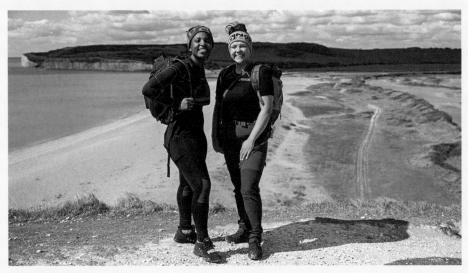

➡️ A guided hike in East Sussex.

diversity crisis. But, the exclusive nature of these careers means that often they don't have the widest representation of different cultures. In fact, conservation is the second least diverse sector after agriculture, and on nine out of ten occasions, I am the darkest-skinned person at any meeting. When you start talking about things like colonialism, people get uncomfortable, but this is a legacy of colonialism. And, especially since women of colour are the ones who are most affected by the outputs of climate change, we really need to be part of the solution.

I was lucky enough to win a place on the RSPB programme. I held a one-year position from April 2022 to April 2023 and there were four of us on the course. The purpose was primarily to train us in conservation skills. Through the traineeships, we learned lots of practical things that are impossible to learn at university. These skills, known as 'tickets', are often

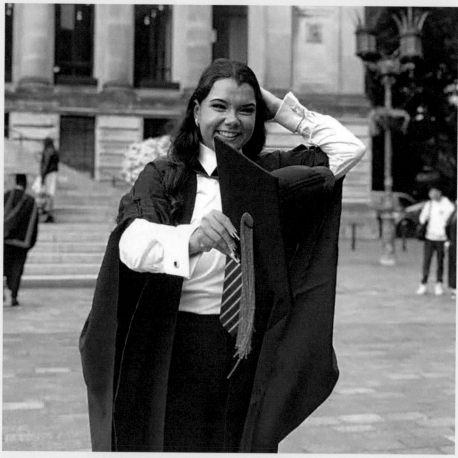

➡ After graduation, I wanted to work in conservation or the environment.

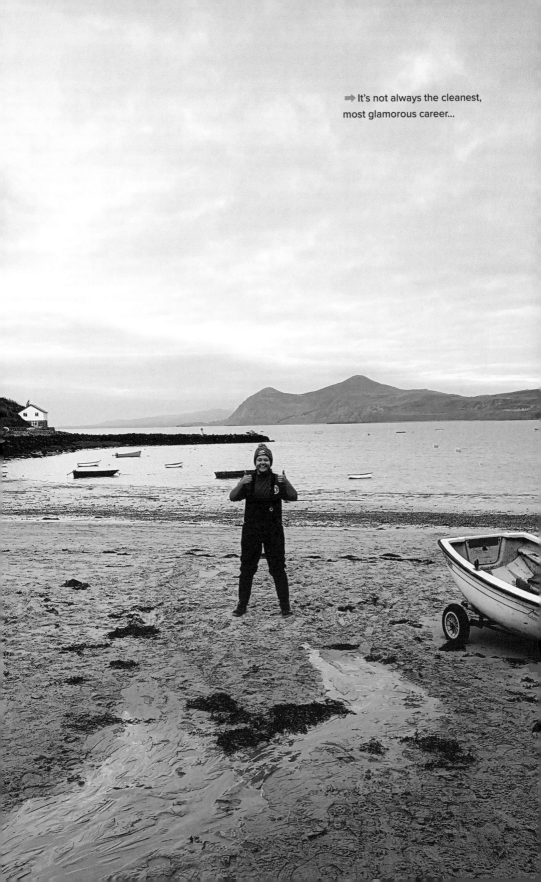

➡ It's not always the cleanest, most glamorous career...

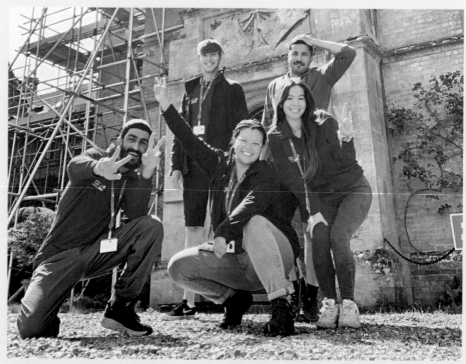

➡ The RSPB program gave me skills I would have struggled to gain elsewhere.

approved by manufacturers and are things you might know if you have grown up on a farm, for example, brush cutting, strimming, and 4X4 and ATV driving. We also carried out fish and bird surveys and helped stranded marine mammals.

I went into this sector to focus on nature, but it's hard when you have to instead focus on the people around you. I actually had a colleague turn around to me early on and say, 'Choose your battles, it takes a lot out of you.' Six months later, I told her I understood what she meant. I've been asked, 'Are you lost?' when I've been out on site in full uniform. I've also been told, 'You don't belong here.' This has spoiled my enjoyment of my role. I wanted to go into nature to have some escape, to appreciate the beauty. I don't want to be looking over my shoulder.

Now my traineeship is complete I'm going travelling. I'm not sure what I want to do long term — after this year I'm a bit hesitant now about conservation as a career. I feel like the sector has a lot of improvement to do. So, for now, I will spend six weeks scuba diving in Mexico, where I will be with people from the local community and scientists involved in monitoring data that is sent to academics. Seagrass and oysters are my area of specialism. I can't wait!

EMPOWERMENT

Patagonia are a brand that do things differently. They have funded us for a 'Hidden Communities' project that addresses the needs of people historically excluded from the natural environment holistically. This might mean addressing ESOL requirements, older women's isolation and the access needs of the less able-bodied, among other marginalising factors. This is a project that has made me really proud. We're taking people into the outdoors, showing them places to enjoy nature, leading hikes and supporting them to do these things.

Crucially, Patagonia are funding this project for two years – enough time for us to really make a difference – and only require light reporting in terms of letting them know what and how we are doing. This is important: it demonstrates that they trust BGH, and it takes away some of the burden of administration. Instead, we can concentrate on our practical work. Sometimes we have to rethink how we do things, too. For example, we've used old-style paper leaflets to publicise this project, rather than relying on online communication, to reach communities who may have less access to computers and broadband.

Patagonia really exemplify the saying, 'work for a cause not applause'. They're well known for being a B corp, demonstrating the highest levels of environmental and social responsibility, and last year, the owner transferred ownership of the company to its workers. They care about the environment and give lifetime guarantees on their goods. They're more like an environmental charity than a clothing brand.

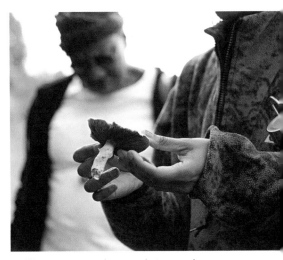

➡ We are encouraging people to experience the natural world.

We are always careful about which organisations we work with, because we have a strong sense of responsibility to our members and we are protective of them. For every negative experience one of them has, that could be a person who would have loved the rural environment lost. Also, word of mouth travels – it could be a whole extended family or group who avoids the countryside in future. This is the exact opposite of what we are trying to achieve.

The Wildlife Trust are a relatively diverse and very concerned organisation, and they have been amazing. We've worked with them on lots of projects, most recently 'Nature Nurtures', which worked with a group of diverse young women to explore the benefits of engaging with the outdoors at Walthamstow Wetlands. They always want to work with us in a meaningful way and their plans are well-structured and with a built-in legacy. This is the kind of work we are keen to do more of in the future.

INSPIRATION

Name:

OGE EJIZU

Age:

35

Profession:

DIVERSITY, EQUITY AND INCLUSION BUSINESS PARTNER

Lives:

ENFIELD, NORTH LONDON

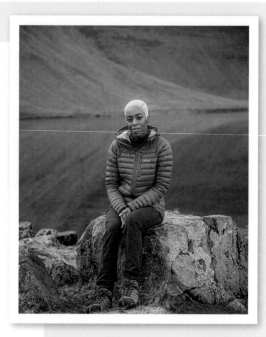

Growing up in the city, I thought that the countryside wasn't for me.
There wasn't any representation. It isn't that there haven't been people of colour who hike, it's more that there hasn't been anybody who has been made visible doing it. Until now, no one has been spreading the message: *Look, you actually* can *do that!*

The countryside wasn't something that ever registered to me as a place you explored. Mixed with that, as a child, I thought that hiking was a white middle-class pastime. I rarely saw anybody like me hiking. I and others therefore associated the outdoors and hiking as something that 'Black people don't do'. I internalised that message and believed it for a very long time.

To make things harder, thanks to the messaging, when you do try to do these things, people look at you like you're weird. Hiking is not encouraged in our communities, and the reasons why are not interrogated.

Despite all this, I started hiking in 2018. Not because I had any desire for it, but mostly because my friend is a persistent nagger and wouldn't take no for an answer. My first thoughts when we went out for walks were,

This is boring, when will we be finished? This is a waste of time! I was very much used to a fast-paced, goal-oriented London life.

The change happened when I allowed myself to be in the moment, when my walking pace slowed, my breathing became deeper and I wasn't holding the tension in my body, and when I actually took the time to notice what was around me. I didn't realise it, but every walk was helping me to be fully present in nature, experience a sense of ease and letting go in my body, and take it all in and enjoy it. But it doesn't mean that every walk is or has been exciting – some have been uneventful or boring and that's fine. Just being out in nature, doing something that detaches me from the business and rush of life, is what I focus on.

My hiking journey began close to London in the Home Counties, in Surrey and around the Woking and Guildford area. It wasn't until my first

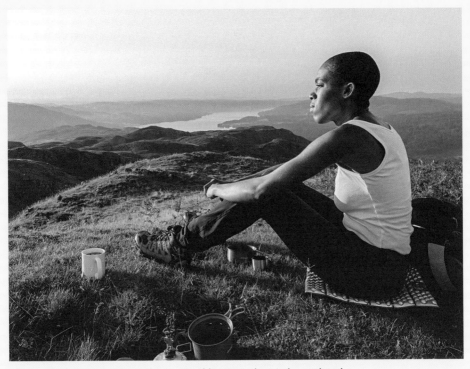

➡ As a child, I never thought the countryside was a place to be explored.

big hike to Dartmoor that my passion for hiking fully blossomed. It was so wild and isolated and such a deep contrast to the urban environment I was used to. Since then, I have been hiking in Wales, Cornwall, the Peak District and the Lake District. Solo hiking is something I also never imagined I would be confident to do but I have now hiked the stunning Pembrokeshire Coast, Gower Peninsula and attempted the Yorkshire Three Peaks in 2021 solo, completing two of these challenges. Although I haven't been to Scotland, it's definitely top of my bucket list. Hiking has given me the opportunity to see just how beautiful the UK is!

Now, I am Regional Leader for BGH. The first hike I led was a two-hour, linear walk in Epping Forest just when the first Covid-19 lockdown eased in August 2020. My thoughts were, *Not many people will want to come out as everything was uncertain, I bet there will be no more than 30 people*. Each time the Underground train pulled into the station, more and more women flooded the car park, and my expectation of 30 people was quickly decimated. I eventually counted up to 100 women. At first, I was overwhelmed. I had to lead them, and make sure I remembered the route. But once we got started, seeing so many women from across generations, hearing stories, talking and spending time together felt amazing. I was in my element!

BGH has given me so much. I have had so many great opportunities through our amazing community. I am now formally trained to safely lead

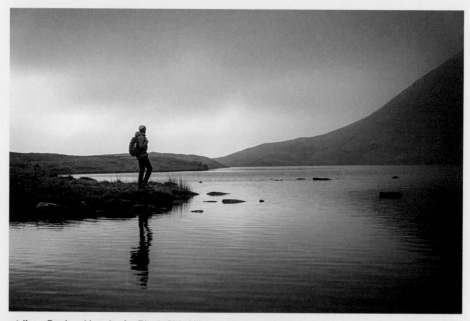

➡ I'm a Regional Leader for Black Girls Hike and in my element.

groups over various terrains. I have completed the Lowland Leader course and Hill Skills and Mountain Skills courses through Mountain Training. Thanks to these courses, I am able to lead groups in relatively flat land and on lower peaks such as those in the Peak District. The next step in my development is to become a qualified Mountain Leader, which can take up to a year to achieve as it's challenging to get enough mountain days when you also have a full-time job. Although it's difficult, I know it will be worth it.

Trying to choose my favourite hike is like asking which one food I couldn't live without! If I had to say which have been most memorable, I would choose Kinder Scout in the Peak District, Helvellyn and Loughrigg Fell in the Lake District. The Lake District was unforgettable, from having an early morning breakfast at the top of Loughrigg Fell to watching the sensational sunrise over a cloud inversion (when you are sitting on top of the clouds and looking down on them) on one of the pikes.

I also love Epping Forest. It's beautiful and it's so unusual to find ancient woodland close to a major world city like London.

The countryside has been a blessing to me. Connecting with nature and learning how to take things slow has done wonders for my physical and mental health. I have seen how hiking has opened up my mind about what I can achieve, how I can push myself beyond what I think I can do, and my ability to get back up and learn from mistakes.

Being outdoors gives me the space and room to just be. There are no expectations or pressure to do anything other than enjoy my surroundings and gather my thoughts. Whenever I'm out hiking, I'm reminded that the mountains were there before me and will be there long after I'm gone. Remembering this helps me put my worries and problems into perspective and just allow myself to be fully present in the moment.

"

BEING OUTDOORS GIVES ME THE SPACE AND ROOM TO JUST BE. THERE ARE NO EXPECTATIONS OR PRESSURE TO DO ANYTHING OTHER THAN ENJOY MY SURROUNDINGS AND GATHER MY THOUGHTS.

"

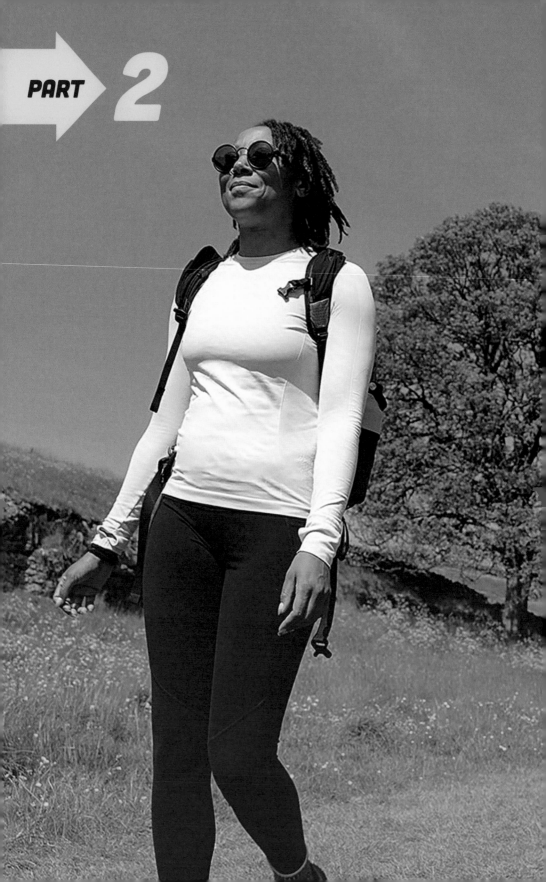

PART 2

HOW?

It's a big world out there and taking your first steps to explore it can feel intimidating. I led my first walk with little experience but a great deal of enthusiasm. And that enthusiasm was key — it helped me find the routes and landscapes which spoke to me as an individual.

To find your hiking mojo, try to block out the expectations and ideas you have picked up from reading about traditional adventurers. There is no need to climb a mountain your first time out! And a route which is beautiful, but not necessarily challenging is absolutely fine.

Similarly, hiking doesn't have to be about fitness goals. You don't have to be completely exhausted and be tracking your 'Personal Best' if all you really want is a gentle stroll in a green environment.

Tuning into your true desires and finding the kinds of adventures which really feed your soul, rather than being sidetracked into what you think you *should* be doing (and what looks great on the 'Gram!) is key. Once you have successfully done this you will reap so many mental as well as physical benefits.

You will learn what gives you a lift. Perhaps it's drinking in a wonderful view, enjoying a picnic after a successfully followed route, or chatting to fellow travellers along the way. And believe me, it's easier than you think to get started. All you need is a bit of basic kit, and some solid advice to follow, and you can begin your outdoor adventure.

And the range of natural environments awaiting your footsteps is extraordinary. The UK is blessed by its countryside and its hills, valleys, rivers, moorland, and coast are waiting to be explored. Not to mention its many species of wildlife. Where will tomorrow find you?

HOW TO BEGIN HIKING

You will have noticed that the outdoor industry is massive, and there is a huge range of equipment available, so this section starts with sorting the 'necessary' from the 'nice to have'. Then I move on to practical advice and start with all t he information you need to get started, from how to pick your first route, to what you really need in terms of hydration and nutrition.

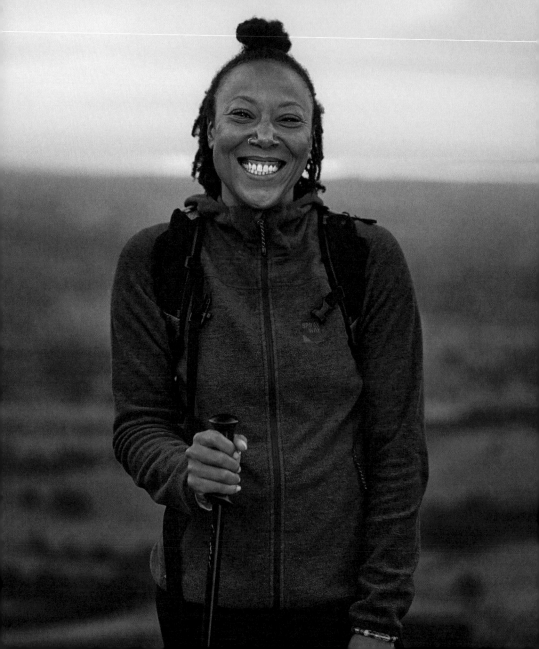

CHOOSING THE RIGHT KIT

Do you know the difference between sweat-wicking, Gore-Tex and antimicrobial fabric? No? Good – it doesn't matter! I know just how confusing and overwhelming it can be – when I first got into hiking, I had to Google half of the kit I was told I needed for a training weekend.

But for beginners, a lot of this is pretty unnecessary. In addition to a comfortable small rucksack (available from about £4 from your local sportswear retailer) and, of course, water and snacks (treat yourself here, you will have earned it and high-quality nutrition is important), there are really only three things you need to get started.

1 HIKING BOOTS

Looking after your feet should be at the very top of your list. It's hard to enjoy anything when you're uncomfortable and in pain. Ideally, so you can deal with all the British weather can throw at you, these will be breathable, waterproof and lightweight with good ankle support. As hiking in rural areas means that you will encounter a variety of different conditions underfoot, you want to make sure you're not likely to twist an ankle or slide off that slippery rock. Look for a pair that are super-light and consider shock-absorbing midsoles for extra cushioning. And remember to BREAK THEM IN!

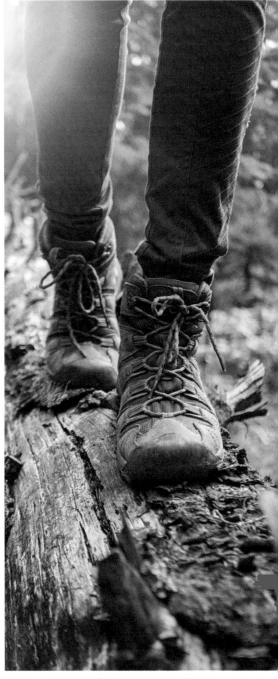

➡ A comfortable pair of hiking boots will get you a long way. © Adobe Stock/Sergii Mostovyi

2 MERINO WOOL TOP

It's counter-intuitive to say you need wool in the summer but cotton absorbs moisture, making your clothes damp and heavy. Then the wind gets up and you're stuck in a damp top and suddenly you're very chilly indeed. The magic words are 'wicking fabric' – this can be synthetic but merino wool is a natural alternative. 'Wicking' means that the fabric draws sweat to the outer layer and dries quickly. So, your top doesn't become saturated with moisture, helping you to stay warm. Clever!

3 WATERPROOF JACKET

But not just any jacket – you're looking for specific features that will make it a permanent addition to your backpack. You need one that's 'breathable', which means you won't sweat in it like you're wearing a plastic bag.

FIRST TIME OUT

Put your water bottle, waterproof and snacks into your backpack and get going! The choice of equipment and walking routes can be overwhelming, so don't over-research. Try not to overthink it, or you might never get out of the door. If it's the middle of winter, you may want to add a warm jumper, hat and gloves to the list above, but none of these things needs to be 'special' – just have look at what you would wear every day.

When picking your route, try to stay local. Exploring your immediate area can be fascinating, and the green spaces on your doorstep can be more beautiful than you ever imagined! Choose somewhere flat with marked footpaths specifically aimed at walkers so you don't have to worry about where you are going or getting lost. For your next adventure, you could try to plan a new route but, for now, you want to break in your boots gently, so don't overdo it. If you do stray too far – perhaps even get dreaded blisters – you'll be glad you stayed close to alternative transport options to get you home.

Remember – experience is the best teacher! And you could always join a group like BGH so that you don't have to worry about the direction you're taking and can simply enjoy your surroundings. You will soon learn what extra items you wished you'd brought – make a note of them. This is you building a kit list. Soon you'll be ready to take on longer and more complex hikes and – just like that – you're a hiker!

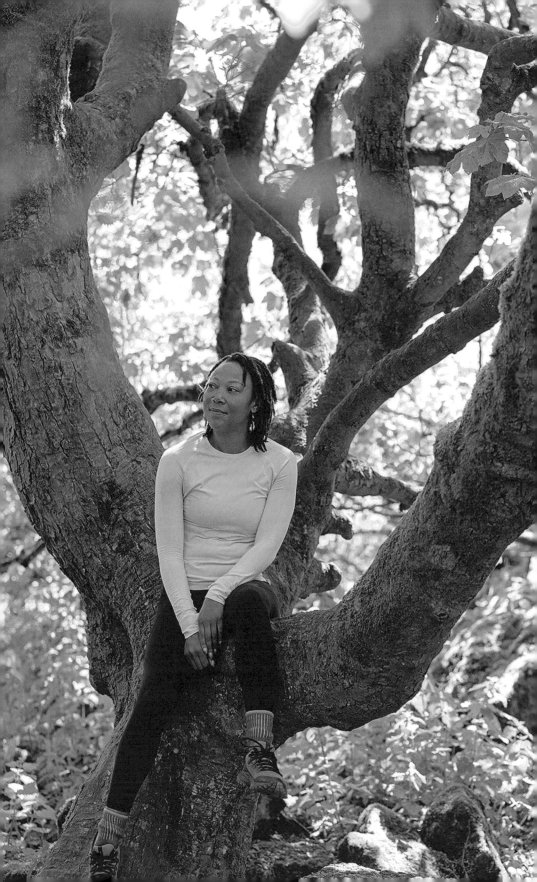

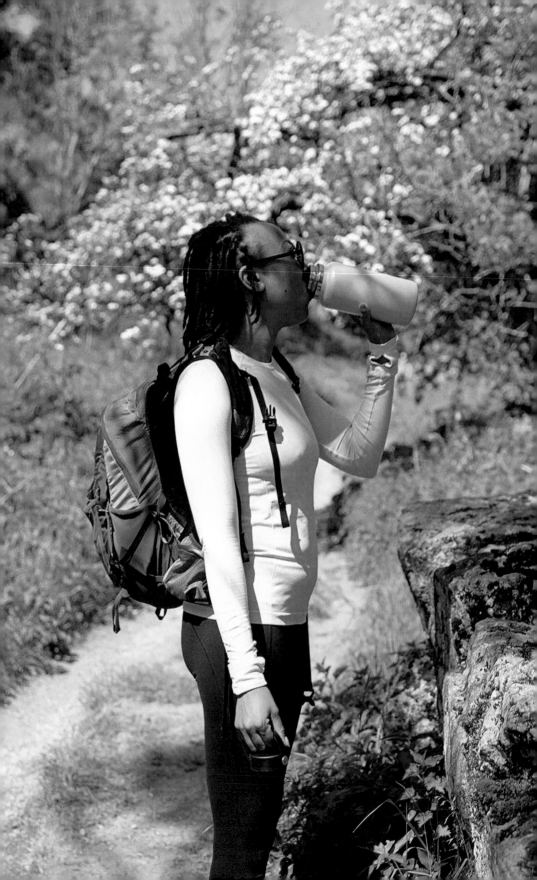

Don't forget a hood – I look for a hood on my jacket that is 'helmet compatible'. This means that if I change my hair so that it has more volume, I can fit my hair under it, with perhaps a hat on as well. I like a peaked hood, too, to keep the rain off my face.

Finally, make sure your jacket is waterproof and not just water-resistant. These terms are not interchangeable! If you get caught in a downpour, you'll learn the difference the hard way, believe me.

NUTRITION

When I first started hiking, I didn't give much thought to nutrition and I didn't know the best foods to support my activities. I underestimated hiking as a workout. We all know that our bodies need carbs, proteins, healthy fats and plenty of fluids for peak performance, no matter what activity we're attempting but for hiking, the best foods are those that release a steady supply of energy to

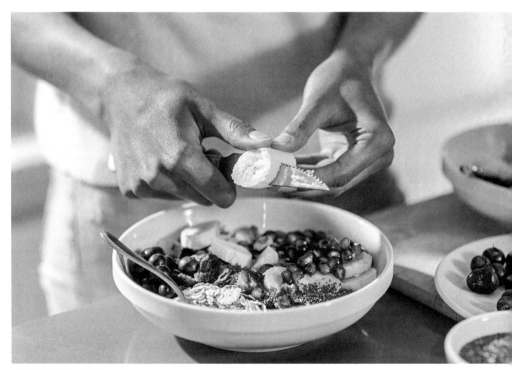

➡ ABOVE: Foods that release energy slowly are a good choice.
© Getty/EMS-FORSTER-PRODUCTIONS
➡ LEFT: Always be prepared. © Photo by Laurelle

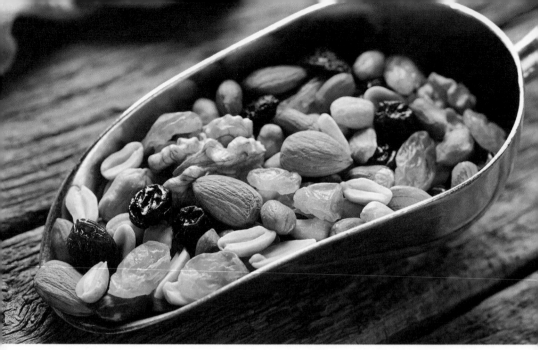

➡ Dried fruit and nuts are great 'on the go' nutrition to carry with you. © Adobe Stock/Ildi

power you through and help your body recover. This is the opposite to the types of food I'd eat when I first set out. I'd grab a McDonald's breakfast on the way and pop a supermarket 'meal deal' in my pack for lunch.

While fatty and sugary foods like these can give you a quick burst of energy, they make you feel lethargic after your blood sugar plummets. And the meal deals just didn't provide enough fuel for the day.

Here's how to feed your body properly so that you are most effective in the outdoors. Nutrition is so important that you should plan your food needs along with your route. The second will dictate the first, with longer, more challenging hikes demanding more calories and liquids.

IT'S TRUE: BREAKFAST IS *THE MOST IMPORTANT MEAL OF THE DAY*

Breakfasts of complex carbohydrates, proteins, healthy fats and fibre – foods that are easy to digest, keep us full and provide long-lasting energy. Wholegrain cereals, oats and calcium-packed dairy foods such as yoghurt are ideal. When it comes to breakfast, you want to wake your body up and stock up on carbs for an instant boost. Studies have shown that eating carbs before a workout improves our performance, allowing us to perform for longer or at a higher intensity, which translates to better adventures. I really enjoy overnight oats with dates and, if I grab breakfast on the go now, it's a granola and yoghurt pot.

SNACKING IS GOOD FOR YOU

In fact, it's essential when hiking. Snacking as you go will help to replace the energy you're burning and will keep both your energy and your mood up. Long hikes need lots of fuel, and if you don't eat enough, you'll soon find your mood plummeting. Hiking snacks need to have the right nutritional balance; you want them to be light yet dense, easy to carry and easy to eat on the move. Try things like trail mixes – nuts, dried fruit and cereal designed specifically to be eaten on hikes

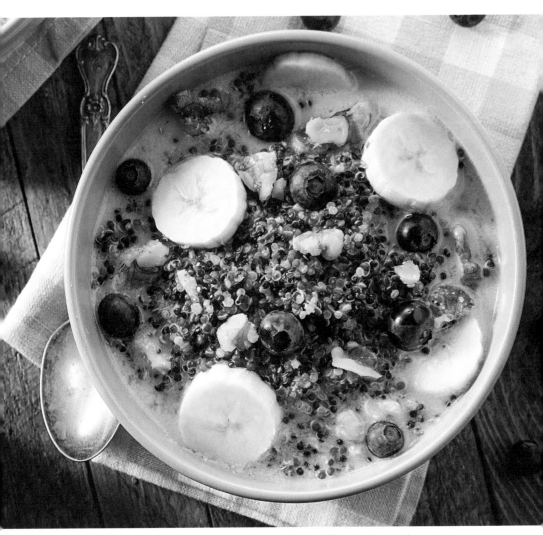

➡ Breakfast is important. Choose complex carbs, proteins and fibre for long-lasting energy.
© Adobe Stock/Brent Hofacker

— as well as cereal and protein bars. Get creative and make your own if you don't like the ready-made versions.

Remember that you're doing this for pleasure, not to punish yourself! I like to stop for cake on a hike if I get the chance, but my go-to treat is ... fizzy laces! I always have a packet of these, and they're fantastic if you need a quick energy boost. That said, generally, high-sugar foods when you're walking are a bad idea, because they can cause sugar rushes and energy drops, but life is about balance and sometimes, all you really want, and need, is a bag of sweets!

> **66**
> ## REMEMBER THAT YOU'RE DOING THIS FOR PLEASURE, NOT TO PUNISH YOURSELF!
> **99**

DRINK AS MUCH AS YOU CAN

Everyone sweats when they exercise; it's not glamorous, but sweating is our body's way of regulating temperature (and also the reason why moisture-wicking fabric is so important). This means you need to top up the fluids lost to maintain your energy, perform at your best and prevent dehydration. Headaches, low mood and even disorientation can result from not drinking enough (and you'll need something to wash those cereal bars, dried fruit and nuts down with).

I always say that water is the best way to hydrate before walking, replenish during a hike, prevent muscle cramps and aid recovery post-trek. When hiking, the rule of thumb is to drink 1 litre (1.8 pints) of liquid every two hours, but how much you drink ultimately depends on what your body needs and hiking conditions on the day. For a short day hike, I usually take 2 litres (3.6 pints). For anything longer or more strenuous, I'd recommend adding electrolytes to replace your salts. If you're collecting water in the wild you'll need a water filter — they're not too expensive and can be a life-saver if you need to travel light.

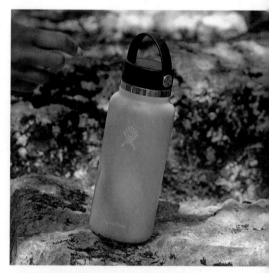

➡ ABOVE: Staying hydrated is essential.
© Photo by Laurelle
➡ RIGHT: Knowing how to use a paper map is vital. © Adobe Stock/Rawpixel.com

NAVIGATION

Navigation used to mean a paper map and a compass, but in today's tech-heavy world, there are many more expensive options. But I believe that the original is often the best: it won't lose power or signal and still deserves a spot in your backpack. Here's what you need to know about finding your way.

HOW TO READ A PAPER MAP

Even though today many of us have smartphones and access to GPS and satellite navigation systems, knowing how to use a paper map is an essential skill. Electronic equipment can lose signal, run out of power, get wet (always carry yours in a zip-lock freezer bag just in case) or simply break down. It's easy to believe that paper maps are a thing of the past, but this simply isn't true.

Of course, you should never go hiking and rely just on your phone's map app, as these don't routinely show footpaths and topographical features. But, even if you have downloaded a more sophisticated version for the outdoors, like the free one available from Ordnance Survey (OS), you can lose signal and end up not knowing how to stay on your route.

Map providers have reported an increase in the sales of paper maps – which is not surprising if you think about it. Not only is a paper map 100 per cent reliable, but it also serves as a souvenir of your trip. It's a physical reminder of your adventures that you can put on your wall and admire if you like.

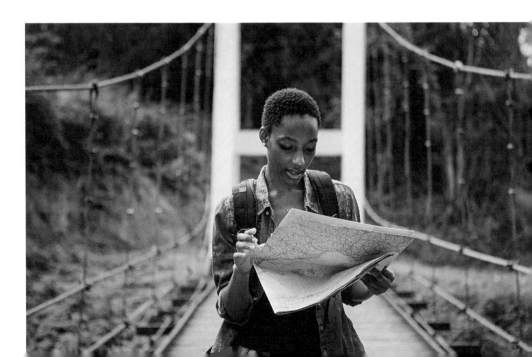

TIPS FOR PLANNING A HIKING ROUTE

• Consider the difficulty of the hike. Some routes are more challenging than others, so it's important to choose a route that is appropriate for your fitness level.

• Consider the length of the hike. Some hikes are short and easy, while others can be long and challenging. Choose a hike that is the right length for your time constraints.

• Consider the weather. If you are planning to hike in the winter, be sure to choose a route that is not too exposed to the elements.

• Consider the terrain. If you are not familiar with the area, be sure to choose a route that is on well-maintained trails.

• Consider the environment. Be sure to leave no trace when you are hiking.

Here is a guide to some simple map reading skills. If you want to take your knowledge further, Ordnance Survey have some fantastic free resources on their website, which go into a lot more detail than I have space for here. These maps are also hugely popular and, if you did any orienteering or map reading at school, it's likely that they were OS. So, I'll assume you're using OS maps, and will refer to the way they're set out and the information and symbols they include in the guide below.

First, invest in a map reading compass (from about £5). Being able to easily find north will make navigation and map reading much easier (and help you make sure you have your map the right way up!).

CHOOSING THE RIGHT MAP: TOPOGRAPHY AND SCALE

For hiking, you'll need a topographical map, like an OS map, which shows detailed information about the kinds of terrain, roads and footpaths, and how steep hills and valleys are. This is quite different from a road map used for driving, where the priority is to show road layouts, whereas the physical landmarks and features in the landscape, such as fields, lakes, forests and hills, are secondary or not marked at all. Tourist maps are no use for anything other than city-centre wandering. They may not be to scale and won't have all the information you need if you want to go for a walk in a city.

The next choice to make is choosing the correct scale. Scale means how much

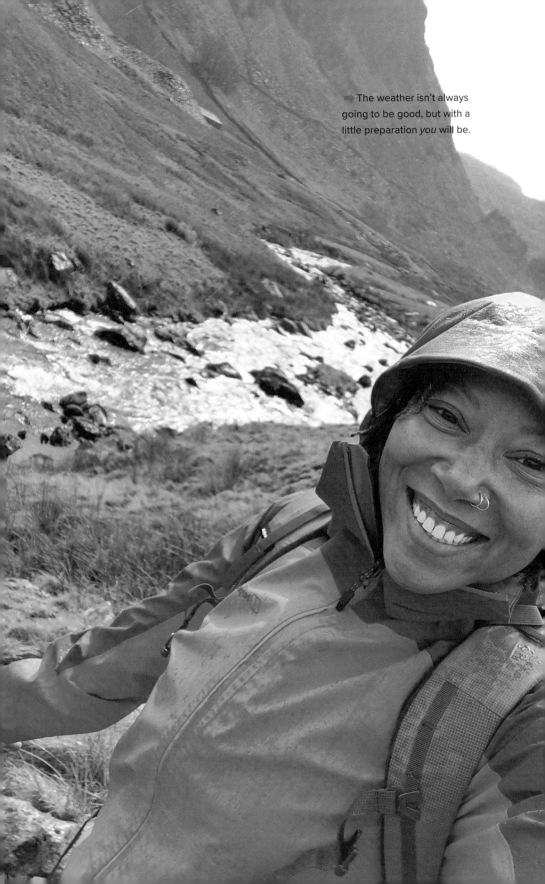

The weather isn't always going to be good, but with a little preparation *you* will be.

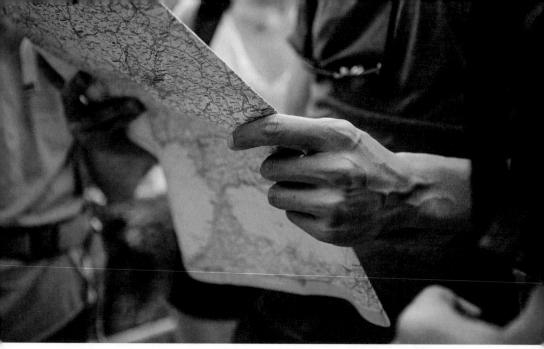

➡️ **A paper map will never run out of power or lose connectivity. © Adobe Stock/Rawpixel.com**

the area on the map has been shrunk down to fit on the paper. It's a bit counter-intuitive that the smaller the area covered by the map, the larger the scale.

OS produce 1:25,000 maps, which is the most useful scale for hiking. 1:25,000 means that every 1 unit of measurement on the map represents 25,000 of the same measurement in real life. For example, 1cm = 25,000cm = 250 metres. This means that 4cm on the map equates to 1km on the ground in real life.

Smaller-scale maps may have a scale of 1:50,000, which means that 1cm on the map is 50,000cm, or 500 metres in real life. So, 2cm on the map represents 1km on the ground.

The map scale of 1:25,000 is usually best for hiking, giving you a very high level of detail – represented by symbols and contour lines, which I explain in more detail below.

GRID LINES AND REFERENCES

What are those squares faintly printed all across the map for? And what do these have to do with the scale? Well, the lines (called grid lines) help you to easily see how far the distance is between two points.

The grids on 1:25,000 OS maps are 4cm wide, and each 1cm = 250m. So, you know that each grid square is the equivalent of 1km across. Diagonally, from corner to corner, the distance works out as about 1.5km.

So, at its most basic, if you count the number of squares between two points, you know how far apart they are. For example, four squares across or up on the map is equal to 4km in real life.

MAP SYMBOLS

There are quite a few symbols on maps that are useful to know. What follows is just a selection of the most important ones, but each map has a legend, which is a key to what each symbol means. But learning some basic ones by heart will save you a lot of time checking the legend and is well worth doing.

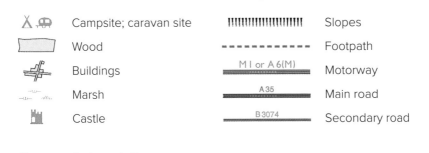

Campsite; caravan site		Slopes	
Wood		Footpath	
Buildings	M I or A 6(M)	Motorway	
Marsh	A 35	Main road	
Castle	B 3074	Secondary road	

Some symbols are letters:

FB – Footbridge   Pol Sta – Police station

PO – Post office   Sch – School

There is a full list of symbols on the Ordnance Survey website.

GRID REFERENCES

The horizontal grid lines are called eastings and the vertical lines are called northings. You can use these eastings and northings to come up with a unique number, known as a grid reference, to pinpoint a location on a map. Lots of walks have grid references to indicate the start and end, and various points along the route.

The most common kind of grid reference is a four-figure grid reference (although six-figure ones are common too). This is worked out by going along the eastings until you align with the bottom-left corner of the square you want – this is your first number. Then go up until, again, you find the bottom-left corner of the square you're looking for – this is your second number.

Remember the phrase 'along the corridor and up the stairs', to remind yourself that the 'easting' is the first two numbers and the 'northing' is the second two.

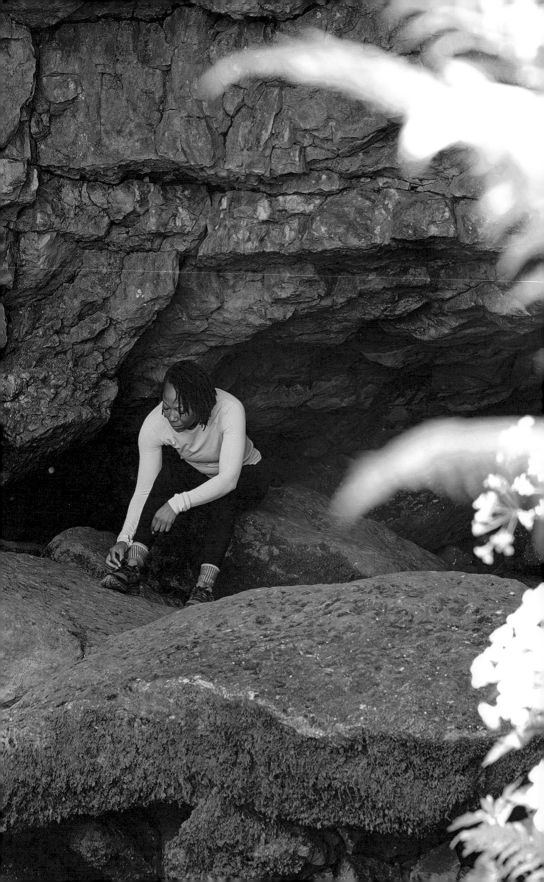

CONTOUR LINES

The topography around the UK is rarely flat. It's covered with hills, mountains, valleys and all sorts of other ups and downs, and this is communicated in maps using contour lines. These are the wavy lines, with numbers next to them. The lines represent the contours or shape of the land, and the numbers tell you the height each line is above sea level. On a 1:25,000 scale map, contour lines are usually placed every 5 metres to show how steep the area is – in really mountainous areas they might be every 10 metres (use your map's legend to check).

The closer together the lines are, the steeper the slope, and vice versa. If the contour lines are pointing in a 'v' shape and they look close together, this will suggest a steep, narrow slope. The opposite of this (a group of lines in an 'n' shape) might signify a decrease in the height.

Contour lines are incredibly useful when planning a route, as you can get a good idea of how steep it will be and

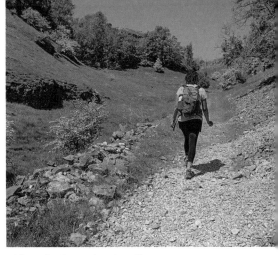

➡ Learning to read contour lines means you can estimate how steep your route is.
© Photos by Laurelle

prepare for it. Adding time on for a slope is important. A helpful guideline is that for every 10 metres of height climbed, you need to add on an additional minute of expected walking time.

The land's contours are the most fixed aspect of a landscape. Trees can be cut down, new paths can be built and old ones become overgrown, walls can be dismantled and streams can change course. What this means is that contour lines are the most reliable features on your map and the first thing you should use to determine your location.

HOW TO PLAN A HIKING ROUTE WITH OS MAPS

1. Go to the OS Maps website or open the OS Maps app on your phone.

2. Zoom in on the area where you want to hike.

3. Click on the 'Create Route' button.

4. Add waypoints to your route by clicking on the map.

5. Once you have added all of the waypoints to your route, click on the 'Save' button.

6. You can then download your route to your phone or computer so that you can follow it offline.

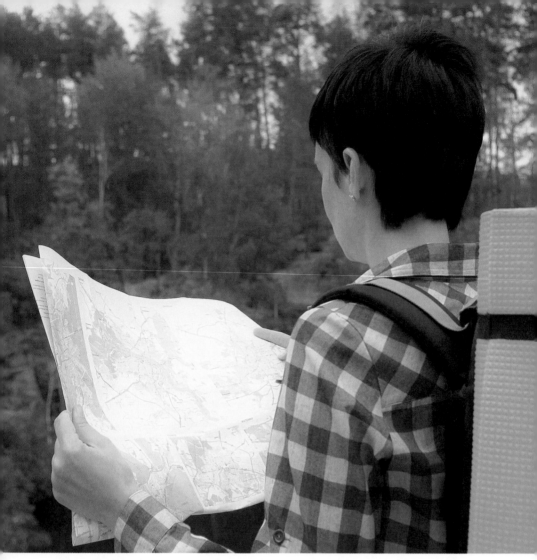

➡ It's unlikely, but if you *do* get lost remember to keep calm and use the landscape to help.
© Adobe Stock/vadosloginov

HOW NOT TO GET LOST, AND ADVICE IF YOU DO

It has happened to all of us. You suddenly think, *Oh no, I don't recognise this path/ headland/field*. Maybe you start turning your map or device this way and that to try to get a bearing and work out where you are. As I showed when I got my group lost, a bit of forward planning can really help to make this scenario a lot less likely. However, should you get lost, a cool head and a bit of common sense will mean you'll get back on track in record time. It's about keeping your wits about you and using the landscape to help you.

TIPS FOR PLANNING A HIKING ROUTE WITH OS MAPS

- Use the 'Layers' menu to turn on different layers of information, such as roads, trails and water bodies.

- Use the 'Search' bar to find specific locations or features.

- Use the 'Zoom' buttons to zoom in and out of the map.

- Use the 'Pan' buttons to move around the map.

- Use the 'Measure Distance' tool to measure the distance between two points on the map.

BEFORE YOU GO

Pack two forms of navigation equipment

A paper map and an electronic app or GPS are the ideal combination. Electronic gadgets sometimes fail, and sometimes, so does our map reading! If you take both, not only have you got a failsafe, but you've got two forms of information to compare, should you find yourself off the beaten path and clueless.

Don't keep your plans to yourself

The most important thing you can do before venturing out is to tell someone what your plans are, where you are going and what time you expect to be back. This is the number one reason for hikers getting into trouble – they are not missed.

Let your friends know, tell your family, even your neighbours. Update your social media. That way, if you don't return on time, people back home will naturally become suspicious and inform the emergency services that there's a problem or even start a search party.

"
AS SOON AS YOU BEGIN TO FEEL LOST - STOP!
"

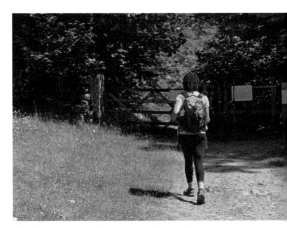

➡ Make sure you let someone know where you're headed. © Photo by Laurelle

ON YOUR HIKE

Notice your surroundings

In the event that you do get lost, remember, if you've been taking pictures along your route, these can be used to jog your memory and to help you retrace your steps. Even if you don't regularly take photos while on your hike, make a mental note of landmarks along your route. It makes such a difference if you do get lost if you are able to spot a distinctive feature – a particular tree or a rock formation can be like a signpost.

Stop, think, plan

As soon as you begin to feel lost – STOP! Moving forwards only makes you feel worse, more panicky and less in control, so stay where you are and try to stay calm. Now, think about your environment – can you remember the last landmark you passed? If so, how far back was it and were you headed north, south, east or west? Try to retrace your steps in your mind.

When you are calm enough to do this, you can start to think of an action plan. Check your phone for a signal

(remember, you may have to move to higher ground to find one). Do you have a whistle on you that other hikers might hear? Check your supplies – what do you have with you? Once you're reassured, you can think calmly about planning a new route before you move on.

What to do in an emergency

If you have an accident or you come across someone else who has and it's a serious situation, you may need to call for help from a mountain rescue team. Here's what to do:

1. Make a note of all the important information:

- your exact location (use OS Locate or the What3Words app)

- the name and age of the person injured and what injuries they have

- how many of you there are in your group

- the phone number you're calling from.

2. Find a spot where there's a decent signal if you can.

3. Call 999 and ask for the police first, then ask for mountain rescue once you've been put through. Stay in the same spot until they call you back.

4. Keep yourself and the casualty (if there is one) warm. You might consider carrying a survival bag or shelter, and a head torch in case it gets dark while you're waiting.

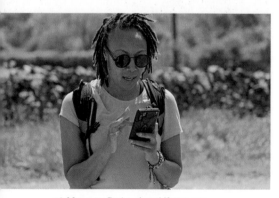

➡ Move to find a signal if you can.
© Photo by Laurelle

CONTACTING EMERGENCY SERVICES VIA TEXT

If you're in an area with bad phone signal you have the option to send a text. However, to use this service you have to register with the emergency services *before* you need to contact them – ie while you're at home.

Here's how to register – it only takes 30 seconds!

• Send a text to 999 with the word 'Register'.

• Read the reply and reply 'Yes'.

• You'll now receive a second text confirming you have been registered – that's it!

If you do get seriously lost, in an extreme case you might have to spend the night in the open, especially if poor weather prevents you from moving on or your rescuers from finding you. If this happens, look for a sheltered spot but without wandering too far from where you began to feel lost. Try to find a space that keeps you out of the rain and other elements as much as possible.

This is why it's essential that you pack extra layers with you too (even if it's a lovely day when you set out). Now's the time to put those layers on. Try to carry high-visibility clothing pieces or a vest, too. This may help rescue services to locate you and certainly can't do any harm!

HIKING HACKS

Hack #1: Know how much sunlight is left

It's much easier to navigate in full sunlight, and as daylight begins to fail it's also much easier to wander off track. So, if you're out hiking, you need to know how many more minutes or hours of sunlight remain. Stretch out your arm in front of you. Every finger width from the horizon to the bottom of the sun represents 15 minutes of daylight.

Hack #2: Know where south is

To tell which direction south is, line up the hour hand on your watch with the sun, then find the point halfway between the hour hand and 12 o'clock – that's south. Of course, you should always pack navigation equipment, such as a compass, but if you ever find yourself without one, remember this trick.

WALKING FOR FITNESS

Hiking is excellent aerobic exercise and, if you are already fit, it will enhance your other training. If you are less fit and want to use it improve your health, it's a great, NHS-endorsed route to improving your fitness: walking briskly can help you build stamina, burn excess calories and make your heart healthier.

The NHS's physical activity guidelines for adults aged 19 to 64 state that you should aim for 150 minutes of weekly exercise. You could start with a brisk 20-minute daily walk during the week and then build up your time and fitness, so you are able to take on longer hikes at weekends.

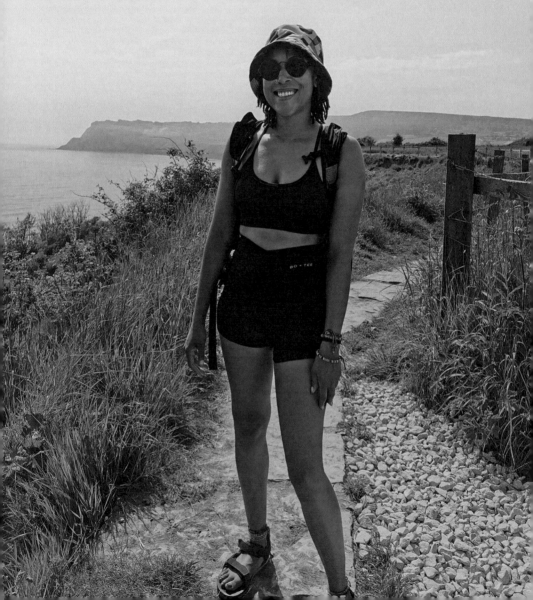

BEFORE YOUR HIKE

One of the easiest and most helpful exercises you can do to keep your knees and legs strong for hiking is static squats. These work the buttocks, front of the thighs (quadriceps), back of the thigh (hamstrings), groin, hip flexors and calves. The quadriceps include important muscles around your knees that help protect them.

Lunges, push-ups and calf raises will also help strengthen your legs and your core (great for maintaining good posture). Just before you hit the trail, perform a brief warm-up routine to prepare your muscles and joints. Simple stretches, leg swings and a light walk can help prevent injuries.

ON YOUR HIKE

Maintain good posture by keeping your back straight and your core engaged. Take shorter strides on uphill sections and use your arms for balance. On downhill sections, lean slightly forwards and engage your core to control your descent. Explore varied terrains — from flat paths to rocky trails and hilly landscapes. This challenges your body in different ways and helps improve your overall fitness.

AFTER YOUR HIKE

After completing your route, perform a cool-down routine that includes stretching major muscle groups. This helps reduce muscle soreness and promotes flexibility. Make sure you are well hydrated, before getting enough sleep to give your muscles a proper chance to recover.

AM I WALKING FAST ENOUGH?

A brisk walk is about 4.8km/h (3mph), which is faster than a stroll. You can tell you're walking briskly if you can still talk but cannot sing the words to a song. You could try using the NHS's free 'Active 10' app on your smartphone. It tells you when you're walking fast enough and suggests ways to fit in some more brisk walking.

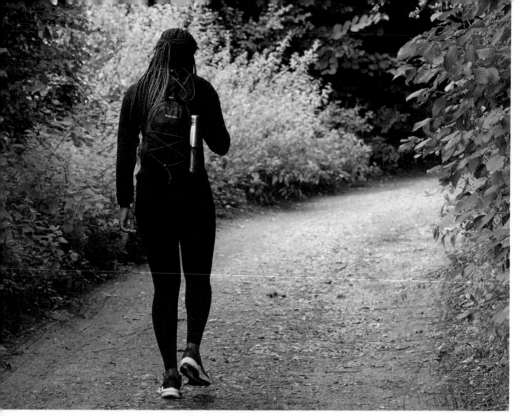

➡️ Make walking part of your everyday routine.

STAYING MOTIVATED

In order to stay motivated, the NHS recommends making walking a part of your daily routine by, for example:

- walking part of your journey to work or the shops

- using the stairs instead of the lift

- leaving the car behind for short journeys

- walking the kids to school

- doing a regular walk with a friend

- going for a stroll with family or friends after lunch or dinner.

You could also listen to music or a podcast while you walk, which has been shown to be beneficial in several ways, including:

- it can take your mind off the effort

- music can get you into a rhythm and help you walk faster

- it can make the time pass more quickly.

However, please do remain aware of your surroundings so that you can listen out for traffic and other people around you.

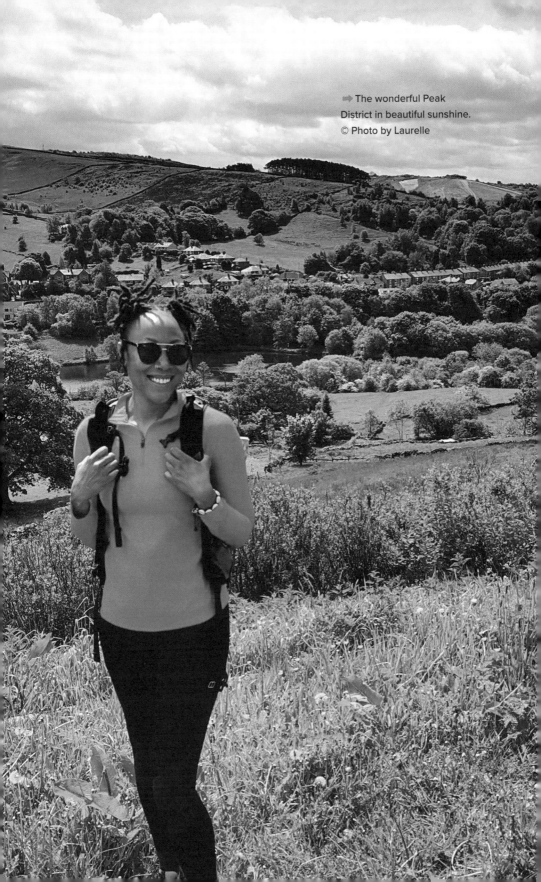

➡ The wonderful Peak
District in beautiful sunshine.
© Photo by Laurelle

TRAINING FOR MORE AMBITIOUS ROUTES

There are times when taking a more structured approach to fitness will pay dividends. Perhaps you are planning a hike that you know you will find challenging, and you really don't want to find yourself exhausted before you've reached the highest point of your trail. Or, you get to the top and you find yourself dreading the descent: your boots feel like rocks, your thighs are burning and your pack has at least doubled in weight since you set off that morning.

In these circumstances, learning to challenge yourself before you get to your destination can mean you really enjoy your hike, so that it's a pleasure rather than an ordeal.

- First, consider building more walking into your everyday life. Increasing your general level of activity can really build fitness and you don't need to pay gym fees or wear special clothes to do it. The NHS has a free app that measures the number of brisk walking minutes you do, and you could work on increasing this day by day.

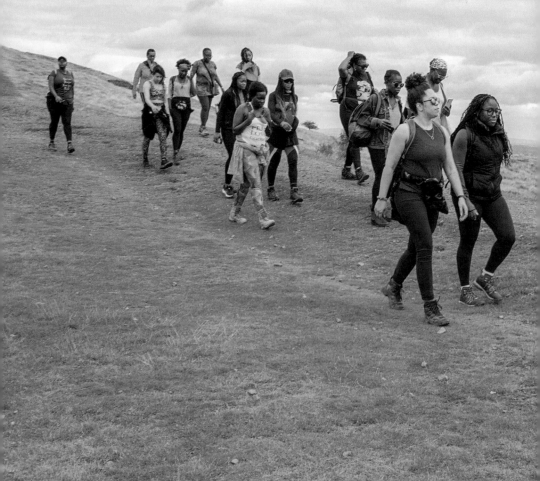

- Take practice hikes with your backpack filled with everything you intend to take. And wear your boots – the extra weight will add resistance to your walking workout and your boots will get nicely broken in.

- Take to the hills – if there's a hill near where you live, practise walking up and down it. If that becomes too easy, increase the number of repetitions or wear your weighted backpack. A smart watch can measure your 'elevation gain' or how far you've climbed vertically, boosting your motivation.

- Finally, if you're shy, use your stairs at home as a virtual mountain (this became a thing among mountaineers during Covid-19 lockdowns when they would share their 'climbs' on social media. Some got to the equivalent of Everest Base Camp!).

AND FINALLY....

Join a walking group – Black Girls Hike would love to welcome you on one of our day hikes or adventure weekends. Walking and chatting with like-minded souls is one of the great rewards of taking to the outdoors – we look forward to seeing you soon!

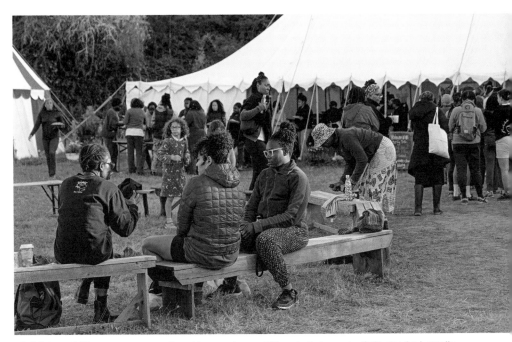
➡ Joining a hiking group easy and enables you to meet like-minded people. © Photos by Laurelle

HIKING ISN'T JUST MOUNTAINS

Hiking isn't only for Black women who live near a national park or Area of Outstanding Natural Beauty (AONB) and have plenty of time. There are lots of different types of hikes available to women of all backgrounds and levels of experience. Most importantly, you don't necessarily have to live in a rural area to enjoy them. Hiking *tends* to be done in nature but if you look closely enough, there's nature everywhere. It might be easier for those who live in the country to step straight out of their front door into natural beauty but urban dwellers can enjoy hiking adventures too.

And there are creative ways to approach hiking that you might never have thought about, which will keep your new hobby fresh and help you stay motivated. One of my favourites is the night hike, with all the sensory stimulation it offers, but there are many others to try, either alone or with friends. Whether you're an absolute beginner looking for a fun way to break in those new boots (try a park hike!) or an adrenaline junkie looking to scale the peaks (see 'Mountain hikes' on page 107) there is always a new style of hiking to try.

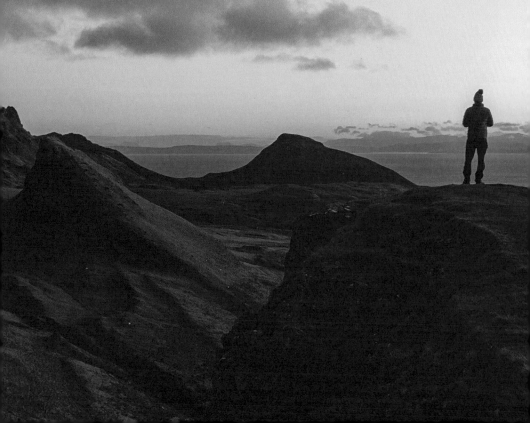

NIGHT HIKE TIPS

- Start your night-time adventures with a route you already know well, so navigation isn't a problem.

- Don't be too ambitious when it comes to distance. Remember, you'll walk slower and need more time for wayfinding.

- Choose habitat and terrain to provide the most interest. Mature woods with cleared paths (look out for bats, badgers or nightingales), open heath, off-road tracks and flat beaches are all good options.

- Avoid anywhere with possible hazards, such as riverbanks, cliffs or steep drops, or anywhere a missed footing, navigation error or not seeing an obstacle might have serious consequences.

- Ideally, start at dusk so your night vision and other senses sharpen as darkness falls.

- Take two torches – a main and a back-up. Take a torch with a red or green light option if possible. You can use these when your eyes have become accustomed to the dark without spoiling your night vision. Wildlife also finds this light less disturbing than white light, so you'll see more creatures.

- Plot your route on a map before a walk, so you're aware of the kind of things you'd rather avoid – or at least be prepared for – whether it's electric fences (beware dairy farms), ditches and stiles, or farmhouses that might have loose dogs outdoors.

- For clear nights, download an astronomy app (such as stellarium-web.org) on to your phone. This will point out all the main stars, planets and constellations for you and may just open up a whole new natural world!

- Carry a map and check your navigation often. In the dark, without familiar visual clues, you can get lost more quickly.

- Temperatures drop faster at night, even in summer, and you'll be moving slower, so carry a warm layer and a raincoat whatever the forecast (you won't see those rain clouds close in).

- If you have to walk on a road, a high-vis vest will be very useful. And put in something to snack on, or a drink, just in case you do become lost.

➡ Take time to enjoy the beauty of nature. © Getty Images/Justin Paget

NIGHT HIKES

Night walking is a brilliant way to refresh your senses and become reacquainted with familiar surroundings in a way that makes them feel brand new. After dusk, the outdoors seems wilder, you feel more adventurous and your senses are dialled up to 11 as your eyes take a back seat and your senses of smell and touch take over.

This isn't just the outdoors without light, but a new space. Trust your senses and your hearing will sharpen to pick up a tawny owl's distant 'keee-wick' or a wood mouse scuttering through dried leaves. Your nose will sniff out the vinegary stink of a fox or the scent of plants such as bladder campion, which only blooms at night. Meanwhile, proprioception (our body's ability to sense movement without thinking about it) will feed back precise information about where you are in relation to the terrain under you and how you're moving over it.

Unless you're lucky enough to live in a remote area that becomes completely dark, your eyes will become super-sensitive to the details around you. The faintest changes in how moonlight illuminates your surroundings, the outline of trees and other landmarks, and the movement of wildlife will all become amplified. This is why night walking can be such a mindful activity – when one sense is reduced, the others take over and your mind is alert to the smallest changes.

PARK HIKES

For beginners, I always recommend a simple hike in a local natural environment. My favourite place to easily access the outdoors is Heaton Park, 8km (5 miles) north of Manchester. It is beautiful at any time of year, enormous (officially the largest municipal park in Europe!) and a circular walk around its perimeter comes in at just under 9.7km (6 miles) – more than a casual stretch of the legs!

For you, it might be your local park, or if you are lucky enough, woodland or forest. And, if you haven't been in your local green spaces since you were a kid (or took your kids), it's time to rediscover them. If you're just starting out, try to stick to the specifically designated routes for hikers to use. This is not only a great way to get outdoors, but it's also a really great way to explore your local area (see 'First time out' on page 78). There's so much that's undiscovered on our doorsteps. Our London group is our most active Black Girls Hike chapter, and they find new and interesting routes to do every week. Our members have been completing the Capital Ring Walk, a 126km (78-mile) route through London's green spaces and nature reserves.

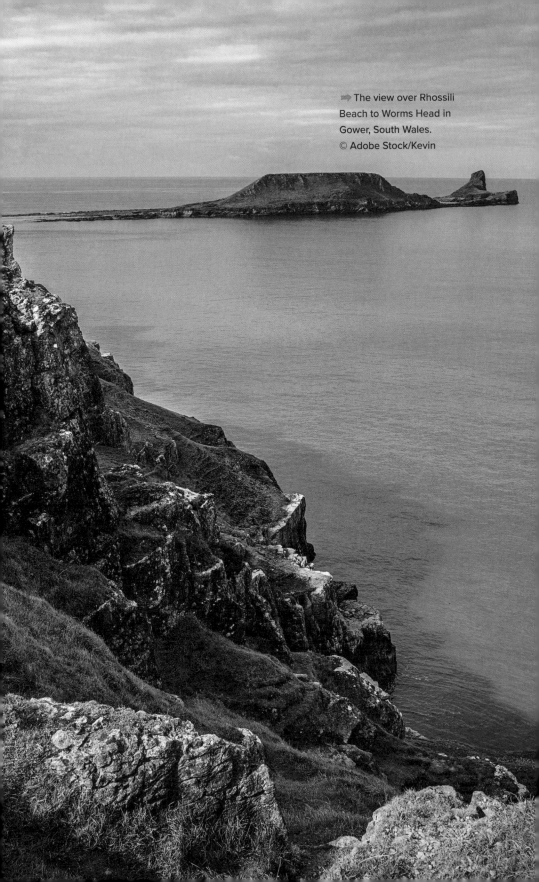

The view over Rhossili Beach to Worms Head in Gower, South Wales.
© Adobe Stock/Kevin

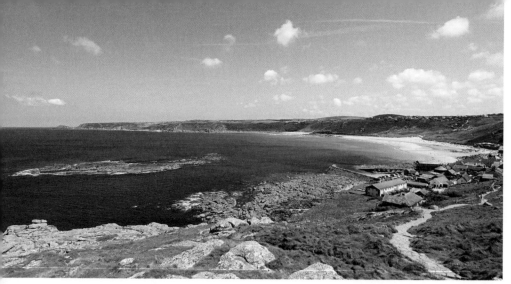

➡️ Sennen Beach in Cornwall. © Adobe Stock/Ian Murdoch

COASTAL HIKES

Coastal hikes provide the perfect excuse for a trip to the beach. In summer, remember to pop in a costume and a towel, and plan a bracing dip after a hike while listening to the waves rushing in and out along the sand. In winter, the sea breeze and the sound of waves crashing against rocks offer an amazing background to a hike. Did you know that there's a 1,400km (870-mile)-long coastal path along the Welsh coast? One of my favourite coastal hikes is a section of the Welsh Coast Path, which runs between Swansea and Port Eynon (for a suggested route along the path, see page 166). It's waymarked and really easy to follow. It can also be split into sections (see 'Long-distance hikes' on pages 110–11 for more suggested multi-day trips).

Hikes like this are a great way to explore the coast without having to worry about navigation. It's much more difficult to get lost when the sea is on one side of you and land on the other! Just remember to stick to the paths and pay attention to signs about erosion and safety near cliff edges.

SUNRISE HIKES

A sunrise hike might just be the most magical way to start your day and I promise, you'll be glad you made the effort. Not just for early birds, what you night owls lose in sleep will be more than made up for as you watch the beauty of the sky at sunrise. Try to find a clear view somewhere high – the top of a hill or by the sea if you can – to enjoy the full power of daybreak. Just make sure that you plan your route, pack your bag and set out your clothes the night before. Nobody wants to be scrambling around for hiking kit at 3 o'clock in the morning!

FINDING YOUR FEET

MOUNTAIN HIKES

If you are feeling fitter, and think it's time for a challenge, a mountain hike is both exhilarating and a workout in equal measure. The extra planning, travel to get to the start of your hike and effort required are all worth it for the satisfaction that comes from being able to say that you've climbed a mountain.

There are plenty of peaks to tackle around the UK, from Yes Tor and High Willhays Tor in Devon to Pen-y-ghent in Yorkshire. For these types of hikes, it's especially important to plan your route – and to take account of the weather. Remember, the weather is often colder and windier in the mountains and conditions can change quickly. That might sound off-putting, but the views are also always better the higher you go, so it's a trade worth making. For mountain hikes, I love the Lake District (consider the hike on page 126 up Scafell Pike, the highest mountain in England). Everywhere you look, the scenery is stunning.

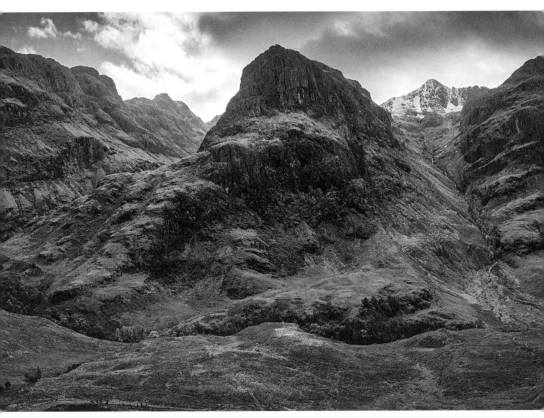

➡ The Three Sisters in Glen Coe, the Scottish Highlands. © Adobe Stock/Ali

GOING A LITTLE FURTHER

When I got lost on the moor with my group of walkers, we should have turned back and retraced our steps. Instead, I led them for hours through strong winds, rain and poor visibility. I had planned for the hike to last two hours but it lasted for four in the end. I've never forgotten how vulnerable we felt against the combined force of the open moor and the elements. Now, I have trained myself to be safe in the countryside and I am an ambassador for Mountain Training, who run BGH's courses for our leaders.

Training is necessary because there is more than just 'common sense' at play here: during the December 2020 lockdown, the Lake District Search and Mountain Rescue Association saw a 70 per cent increase in call-outs to distressed people attempting to enjoy the national park. Most of these rescues, which are carried out by volunteers, could have been avoided had the walkers taken a few simple precautions.

Nature is beautiful and varied, and provides the ultimate mindful activity, as you can only travel as quickly as your legs can carry you, leaving plenty of time to disconnect from your everyday life and bathe your mind in the natural environment. However, if you plan to extend your adventures out of the managed environment of your local park or green space and into the open wilderness, planning will become key.

The first thing to stress is that you should extend the distance of your hikes in stages: this is not a competitive activity, there is nothing to prove here. Plan to walk just a little further than before and follow the tips below. Also, consider doing a course in orienteering (there are online ones available) so you can navigate using a paper map and compass in case you lose network coverage on your mobile phone (see also the chapter on Navigation on pages 85–95).

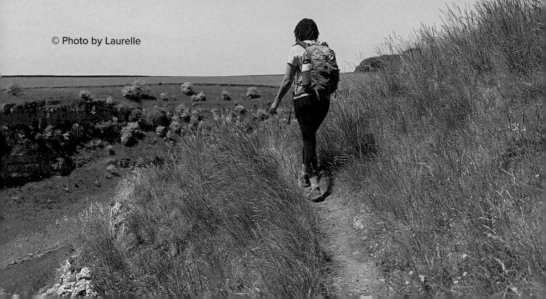

LONG-DISTANCE WALKS ACROSS BRITAIN

Hadrian's Wall Path – 135km (84 miles)

Where: Starts in the fringes of the city of Newcastle in Wallsend, and ends in Cumbria on the Solway Coast, with a variety of trails, from gentle to hard.

Highlights: The variety of landscapes to marvel at, from Roman forts and settlements to beautiful beaches.

The Thames Path – 298km (185 miles)

Where: This route runs from the source of the River Thames in Trewsbury Mead, Gloucestershire to the Thames Barrier in Woolwich, London.

Highlights: See London from a new perspective and follow in the footsteps of Charles Dickens.

The South Downs Way – 159km (99 miles)

Where: This is known as a gentle route, which begins in the beautiful historic town of Winchester and ends in elegant Eastbourne, taking in open countryside, cliff-top paths and sea views.

Highlights: The Seven Sisters Country Park for the classic view of the iconic white cliffs.

The Coast to Coast Walk – 293km (182 miles)

Where: Devised by fell walker Alfred Wainwright, you could walk across the width of England, from St Bees in Cumbria to Robin Hood's Bay in North Yorkshire, taking in iconic Lake District lakes and fells, including Ullswater and Helvellyn.

Highlights: Patterdale, Cumbria, which sits at the southern end of Ullswater, but all of it is gorgeous. Wainwright was a master.

South West Coast Path – 1,014km (630 miles)

Where: The longest national trail in the country stretches from Minehead in Somerset across the coast of Exmoor to Penzance, before turning back on itself and ending in Poole harbour in Dorset. There are hundreds of shorter walks to choose from along the trail.

Highlights: The lovely seaside resort of Ilfracombe. From here, you can walk to the fantastic surfers' beaches of Woolacombe and Croyde.

Offa's Dyke – 285km (177 miles)

Where: Named after, and often following, the spectacular dyke King Offa constructed in the 8th century, this is Britain's longest ancient monument, crossing back and forth from England into Wales. It links Sedbury Cliffs near Chepstow, on the banks of the Severn estuary, with the Welsh coastal town of Prestatyn on the Irish sea.

Highlights: The trail connects three Areas of Outstanding Natural Beauty – the Clwydian Range and Dee Valley, the Wye Valley and the Shropshire Hills.

LONG-DISTANCE HIKES

As you get more experienced and start doing longer trips, you may want to spend more time on the trails. Using hiking as a method of transport like this, walking from point to point along a longer route, can be extremely rewarding, and turn a day trip into a proper adventure holiday. But where do you start?

Don't get carried away with what you think you should carry. If you're not camping, then you need little more than your day sack with a couple of extra changes of clothes. On your first overnight jaunt, it's easy to believe you'll require everything (including the kitchen sink!) just to survive. In fact, you probably need less than you think. Most of the established walking routes in the UK have plenty of villages and towns along the way, where you can stock up on food and snacks, fill water bottles and rest.

If you do want to camp, give it careful thought, and remember it is entirely up to you. There are glory-hunting outdoors people online who would have you believe that unless you travel self-sufficiently, carrying everything you need so that you could wild camp anywhere and be 'self-supported', then you are not a proper adventurer. But, as ever, it is your choice of how wild you want to go, and what you have the tolerance for. Remember that there are glamping sites, too, and that many campsites have extremely good facilities.

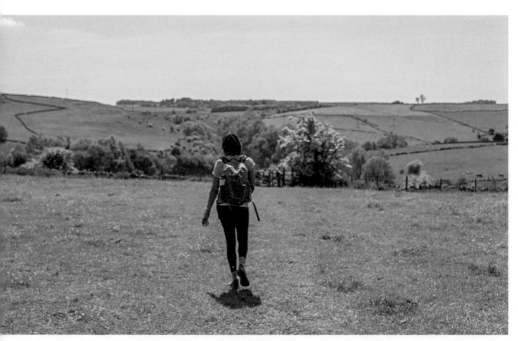

➡ Completing a long-distance hike is deeply satisfying. © Photo by Laurelle

FINDING YOUR FEET

A CAMPING CATASTROPHE

On our first multi-night trip, my friend and I took the train from Manchester to Swansea. We planned to do 9–13km (6–8 miles) a day on a route we'd selected in advance in South Wales. We set off from Swansea really optimistically, carrying our homes on our backs. We made it to Mumbles Head, passed Caswell Bay and walked on to Port Eynon.

But, almost as soon as we started walking, I realised that my backpack was too heavy. My boots were a 'Barefoot' style, and I hadn't done any long walks in them. They're supposed to offer your foot lots of flexibility, but when you first wear them, you can get pain from the muscles you've never used before. I started off aching, then got a massive blister on my toe. At this point, this was ruining my experience and I really didn't want to go on.

When we got to Port Eynon, we fortunately met a lovely woman who helped us – she gave us a lift to her house and let us camp in her back garden. She even gave us a hot dinner! Laughing, she weighed our backpacks – they were 30kg (66lb). We had carried everything – including endless porridge and quinoa. That food was so unappetising when we were tired and hungry. We also took a stove, pans, utensils, even a chopping board!

I'd saved money on my sleeping bag – and saved on warmth, too. So, to add to my misery, I was absolutely freezing at night. Needless to say, after our night with a good Samaritan we headed home from our trip early.

When I look back at our adventure it still makes me smile. I must also say that for that early hike, all of my equipment was from my local sports shop and most of it (other than the sleeping bag!) was absolutely fine. Today, I have mostly top-of-the-range kit that is gifted to me by brands I work with, but the difference isn't that massive. You really don't have to spend a fortune to be comfortable.

If you are feeling adventurous and do decide to camp, then using established campsites is advisable, as the law around camping wild is complex. You will need to carry the extra weight of a lightweight tent, sleeping bag and mat/self-inflating mattress. The upside is that this option will probably save you money, especially compared to booking overnight accommodation in advance (which is advisable on popular routes and during school holidays).

Remember, though, that if you are walking 9–16km (6–10 miles) a day (a reasonable range for your daily hikes), you will appreciate a proper bed and a hot meal much more than you would after a normal day at work. And fatigue can be cumulative – by day four you might feel much less willing to rough it than you did on day one!

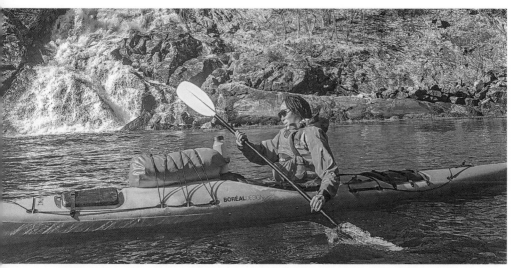

➡️ There are a huge range of activities open to hikers who want to try something new.

ADVANCED ADVENTURING

BGH runs Mountain Skills training weekends for our leaders. The course is aimed at people with some walking experience who want to explore more mountainous terrain and develop their confidence. Our leaders spend two days on the fells, team building and learning everything I didn't know when I got my group lost on Saddleworth Moor!

We looked at developing the key skills needed to explore the outdoors safely, such as planning, navigation, essential clothing and equipment, checking and understanding weather forecasts, group management and emergency procedures.

But if you're new to hiking, this would probably be too complicated. For you, I'd recommend a beginner's navigation course. This will teach you how to read a map and use a compass so you can safely navigate without a mobile phone or GPS connectivity. Being able to plan your own hikes is also really exciting and offers endless possibilities. BGH courses are conducted by Mountain Training. Have a look at their website, and of course come and join Black Girls Hike on one of our next adventures. After your first step, the sky's the limit.

> **DON'T GET CARRIED AWAY WITH WHAT YOU THINK YOU SHOULD CARRY.**

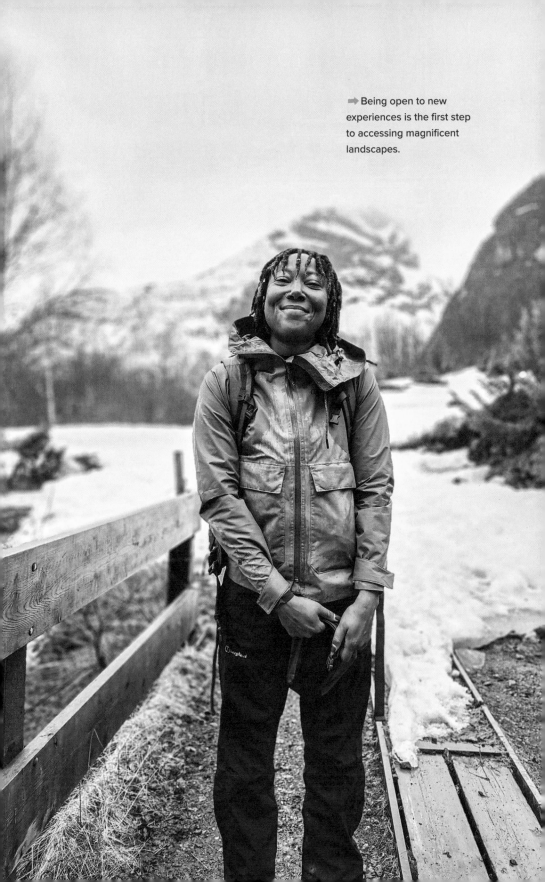

➡️ Being open to new experiences is the first step to accessing magnificent landscapes.

HOW TO BE SAFE AND RESPONSIBLE

I have been keen to emphasise the ease and simplicity of hiking. Nevertheless, the outdoors does have dangers, especially if you go off into remote areas, or are out in the winter at altitude. What follows is sensible advice for keeping you safe, and the natural environment unspoiled.

STAYING SAFE IN THE OUTDOORS

- Always let someone know where you're going and what time you expect to be back. This is particularly important if you're hiking solo.

- If you're tackling a long walk, especially for the first time, plan 'exit' points along the way where you can bail out if you need to.

- Check weather conditions and take notice of Met Office warnings. We've all seen rain and cloud smother a beautiful sunny day, but at altitude the process is faster and more unpredictable. We are lucky here in the UK because, although the weather can change in an instant, on the upside, we don't experience much in the way of extremes.

- Take a proper paper map with you or download the OS Maps app. This will enable you to download routes that you can access offline in case network coverage is patchy.

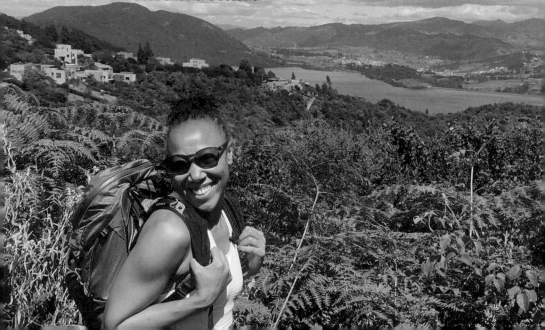

EXTRA KIT

- Consider packing a first-aid kit. These are cheap and easily available online or from chemists.

- In hot weather, you'll need a sun hat, sun cream and sunglasses.

- In the winter, a head torch and batteries may be useful.

- A whistle and survival bag are great to have, just in case.

- A waterproof baseball cap is useful for spectacle wearers.

- Remember that strong winds can be a hazard, and lead to rapid cooling. Make sure you have a hat and gloves.

- Invest in a waterproof (not showerproof) jacket and trousers.

- Take an extra fleece or jumper: plan to keep warm using several thin layers, rather than one thick one (sometimes called a 'base' and a 'mid' layer).

- Carry a high-vis vest, so you can be seen more easily in an emergency.

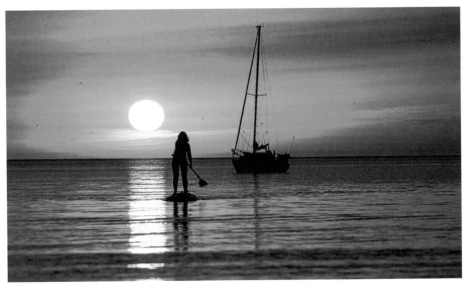

➡ ABOVE: Paddleboarding into a perfect sunset. © Charlotte Graham
➡ LEFT: Hiking outside Bogotá.

WHERE CAN I GO?

The history of our 'right to roam' in the countryside

Historically, there has been a lack of diversity in outdoor spaces more generally, and the British countryside in particular. Numerous factors have contributed to this (many of them, such as socioeconomic disparities, cultural barriers, lack of awareness and limited representation, have been discussed elsewhere in this book).

However, the right of all UK citizens to explore the countryside was fought for over generations. This 'freedom', like many we take for granted today, was for hundreds of years deeply controversial.

The right to roam in the UK refers to the legal concept of public access to privately owned land for recreational purposes. It allows individuals to explore and enjoy certain areas of the countryside, including mountains, moors, heaths and common land. The history of the right to roam in the UK can be traced back to several key developments:

1. Enclosure Acts: In the 18th and 19th centuries, a series of Enclosure Acts were passed in the UK. These laws meant that what had previously been 'common land' and open fields accessible to all were fenced or policed by landowners who used their right to restrict public access to previously available areas.

2. As a result, people living in industrialised and polluted cities could only look up at the wonderful greenery and fresh air on the heaths and moors towering above them, and were not allowed to walk on them.

3. Beginning in the 1880s, people had tried to pass laws in Parliament to give access to mountainous areas. These laws failed to come into existence because many MPs were landowners who wanted to maintain their grip on the countryside.

4. By the 1930s, the 'right to roam' movement had been formed, with the aim of gaining access to the countryside for ordinary people. They would organise 'mass trespasses' on to private land. Walkers would sometimes physically fight with landowners' staff to avoid being chucked off the land.

5. The most famous mass trespass took place on Kinder Scout in the Peak District in 1932. Six hiking leaders were arrested, and one served four months in prison for his 'crime'. This sparked public support and by the early 1950s, national parks began to be established, modelled on Yellowstone in the USA.

6. National parks now make up to 12 per cent of Britain's land surface and more than 3,220km (2,000 miles) of public right of way. They are not owned by the state: the majority of the land is private, but they are protected for all of us to enjoy.

© Photo by Laurelle

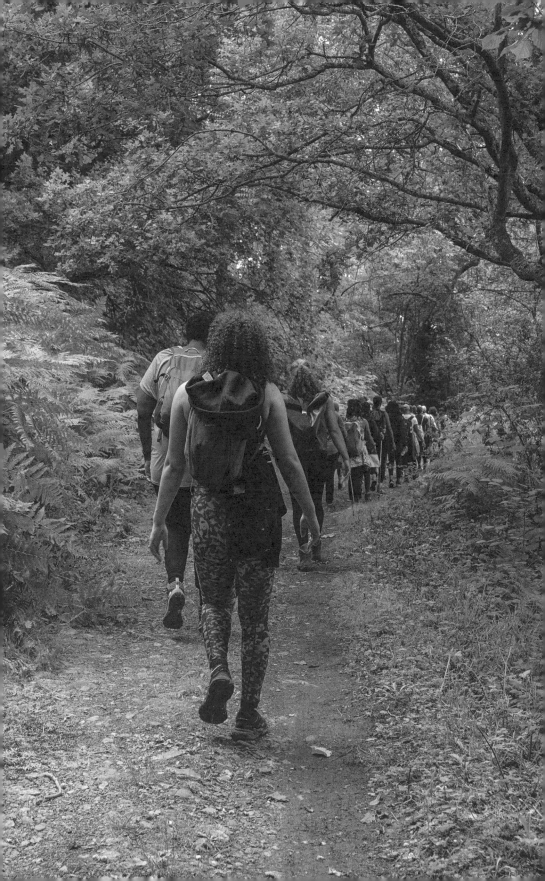

RESPONSIBLE HIKING

Hikers love the countryside they move in, and are, on the whole very responsible travellers.

Following basic guidelines when visiting outdoor spaces means using it sustainably, so that the environment is preserved and the beauty of the landscape is maintained.

• Stick to designated paths and tracks. Use established paths and trails to minimise your impact on the environment. Avoid trampling vegetation or creating new paths that can lead to erosion.

• Leave no trace. Take away all your litter and dispose of it properly in designated bins. Do not leave any waste behind, including food scraps or packaging. Leave the area as you found it or even cleaner.

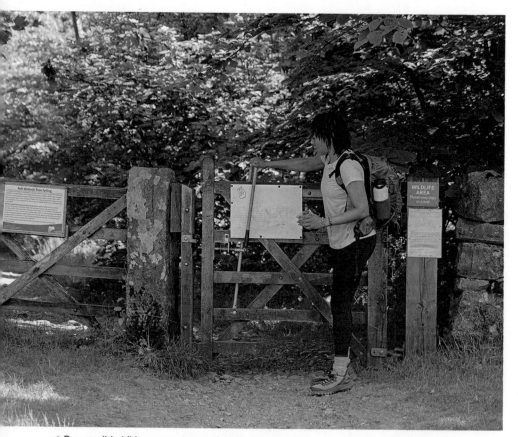

➡ Responsible hiking means protecting the environment and respecting access restrictions.
© Photo by Laurelle

- Respect wildlife. Observe wildlife from a distance and avoid disturbing or feeding animals. Do not pick or remove plants, flowers or other natural resources.

- Follow the countryside code. Familiarise yourself with the specific guidelines and regulations of the area you're visiting. Some places may have specific rules to protect sensitive habitats or wildlife.

- Keep dogs under control. If you're bringing a dog, keep it on a leash where required, and always clean up after your pet and dispose of it responsibly. Be aware of any restrictions or areas where dogs are not allowed.

- Be considerate of other visitors. Respect the peace and tranquillity of the countryside by keeping noise levels down. Yield to others on narrow paths and avoid overcrowding in popular areas.

- Support local businesses. Contribute to the local economy by using local accommodations, eating at local restaurants, and purchasing goods from local shops. This helps sustain the local community.

- Educate yourself. Learn about the local culture, history and traditions of the area you're visiting. Understanding and appreciating the local context can enrich your experience and foster respect between residents and tourists.

- Be mindful of access restrictions. Some areas may have limited access

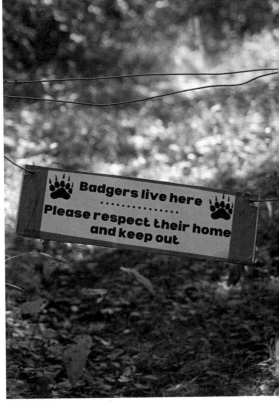

➡ Specific rules protect different habitats.
© Photo by Laurelle

or specific rules due to conservation efforts, nesting seasons or other factors. Respect restrictions to protect sensitive habitats or wildlife.

- Consider sustainable transport options. Whenever possible, use public transport or carshare to minimise your carbon footprint.

For more information, the Countryside Code can be downloaded here: www.gov.uk/government/publications/the-countryside-code

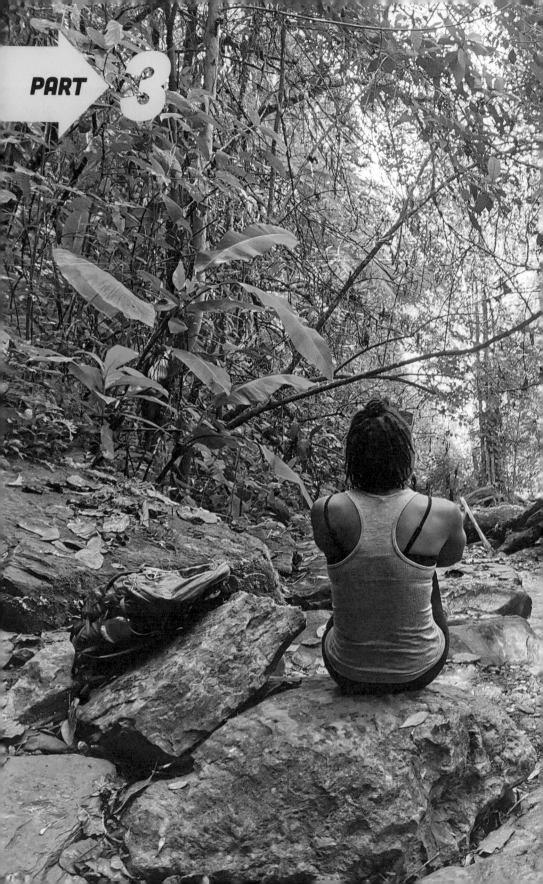

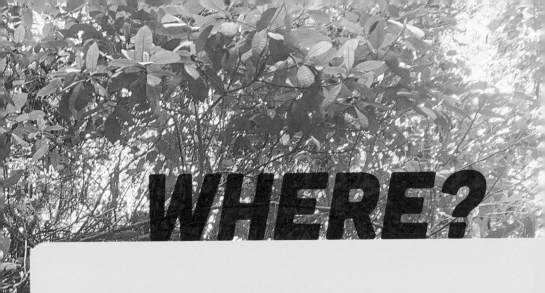

PART 3

WHERE?

TIME TO GET HIKING!

What follows (in alphabetical order) are some of my favourite British walks, most of which have been chosen with beginners in mind. There are a variety of difficulties and terrains here, with urban walks as well as coastal, moorland and parkland all represented. There are some challenges, too – Glencoe is a high and wild, but a classic Scottish adventure. Similarly, Scafell Pike is a well-known challenge. It's not so difficult it couldn't be attempted by a fit beginner (perhaps with a more experienced companion) but it may be that it becomes a goal for you to work towards, offering the achievement of climbing the highest mountain in England.

Feel free to choose whatever suits you, is accessible and matches your sense of adventure. Hiking is not a competitive activity. It's completely OK to stick with the routes and the landscapes you are comfortable with. But equally, perhaps when you become a little bored with your favourite hikes, it's fine to seek out more challenging routes.

You will find some walks are part of much longer national trails, such as Port Eynon to Rhossili, on the Wales Coastal Path. Like other trails that are part of longer routes, if you live near to or particularly enjoy this landscape, you might want to explore it more. You could use your beginner walks as a basis for repeated visits or to work towards a multi-stop trip. Recording your achievements and sharing them with other members of your hiking group (perhaps via

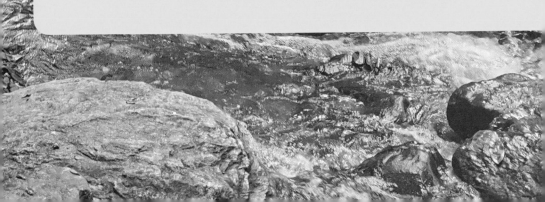

the BGH Facebook page!) is a way of building your hiking network. Some of the well-known routes described here will be an excellent conversation-opener.

Similarly, a multi-stop trip is an exciting prospect and surprisingly social, even if attempted alone. You will meet other hikers who are exploring the trail, and you will start to make friends along the way. Some of my best conversations have come as a result of the camaraderie and sense of common purpose you develop while hiking along a popular route.

These include the stunning Ravenscar circular walk in North Yorkshire, which covers part of the famous Cleveland Way, which starts in Helmsley and ends at Filey Brigg, around 175km (109 miles) later. This walk allows you to take in a wonderful range of North Yorkshire scenery, from wild moorland and stunning sea views from the rugged cliff tops (you might be lucky like me and see a seal in the water – they congregate to breed on the cliffs below Ravenscar).

Similarly, Sennen Cove and Land's End form part of the South West Coast Path, which runs right around the South West coast of England. These long-distance paths criss-cross the country, and you probably live near one, or can easily get to one. They are promoted by National Trails, and there are 16 of them designated by central government, covering around 4,023km (2,500 miles). They are an important symbol of our hard-won freedom to move through the country on foot.

All this is not to say that urban walks cannot be equally satisfying. The Thames Path covers the whole length of England's longest river, the Thames, from the Cotswolds to the sea. The section through the centre of London is perhaps the cheapest and least congested way of enjoying hundreds of cultural landmarks. As an alternative, I have included the less well-known Grand Union Canal walk through London, passing as it does through several recently redeveloped

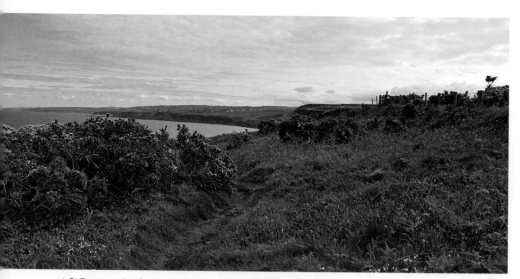

➡ St Bees on the Cumbrian Coast. © Adobe Stock/dejavudesigns

FINDING YOUR FEET

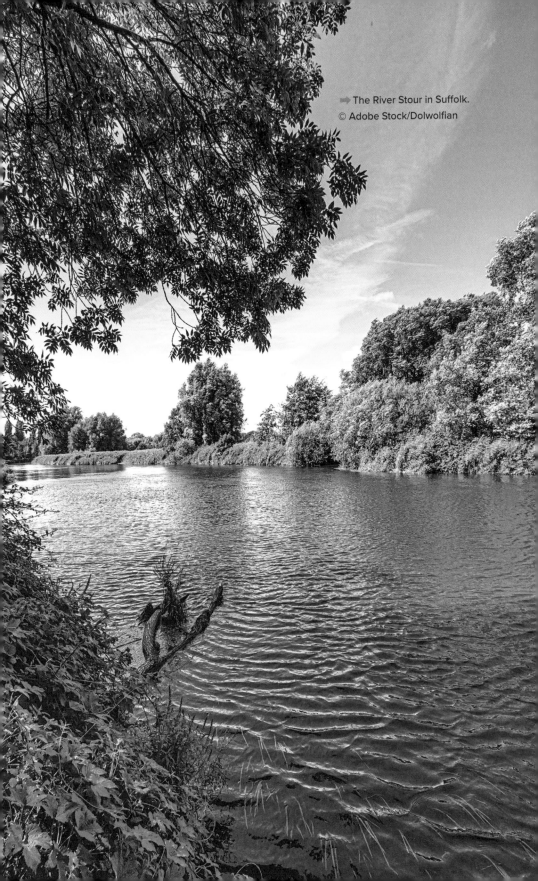

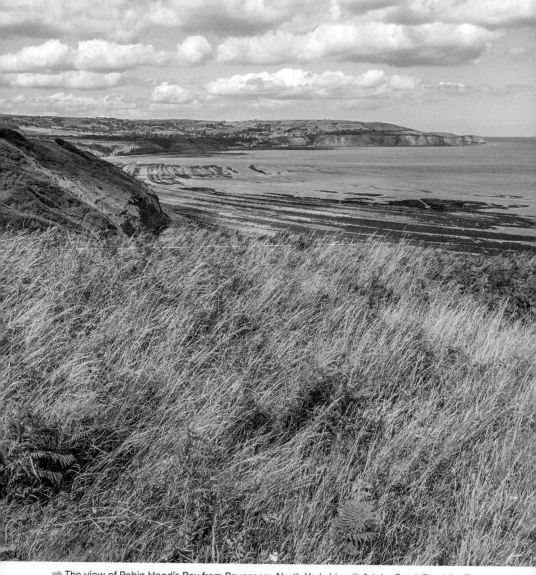

➡ The view of Robin Hood's Bay from Ravenscar, North Yorkshire. © Adobe Stock/RamblingTog

and less-visited areas of the capital, such as King's Cross and Limehouse Basin.

Other routes are included because they offer a particular flavour of a region. From the ancient and end-of-the-world atmosphere offered by the St Bees circular in Cumbria, to the introduction to the South Downs and the maritime culture of Newhaven offered by the walk from Southease, there is something here for everyone.

Please note that you should take a map with you – these descriptions are here to give you a flavour of the hikes, but they are not detailed enough to use alone. Besides, landscapes, access rights and even the weather change the appearance of the landscape and to some extent may alter your route.

THE INTERVIEWS

Once you start getting outdoors you'll notice the sheer range of activities you'll encounter, on land and in the water, underground ... in fact, all around you. Some of these, such as surfing and paddleboarding, are relatively familiar, while others, like mountaineering and caving, are by their nature more obscure. But all of them have required brave and inspiring women to open the door to wider access to these sports, and many of them are interviewed here. These women have fought for themselves and for marginalised groups – whether by race, faith or disability – with a fearlessness that is inspiring.

It was a wonderful adventure to bring these voices together, and it's my pleasure to include them throughout this section. The women are of vastly differing backgrounds, ages and approaches, yet their stories often echo the same themes. They all say there was a lack of representation in their activity and they had to reach out, via social media or blogging, to find others who already did their activity or wanted to join in. More often than not, this led to a community clustering around them, as they found other people who shared their enthusiasm.

As they found their people, they often found their voice. They realised that things needed to change to make their activity more inclusive, so that people who wanted to take part now didn't have to go through what they had to. So, the women here are not just excellent in their fields, they are also community leaders, activists and role models, and some are influencing policy-making at the highest levels.

They nearly all speak to the powerful influence of the natural environment on their mental, physical and spiritual health. They all want to spread the word that the outdoors, and the benefits to be found there, belong to everyone, even if it feels, at first, that this might not be true. And, on the way to their achievements, they have all broken through their own personal barriers, as well as the structures and organisations that have limited the participation of people like them in outdoor pursuits.

I am so proud of these adventurous women, and I think you will be too.

> **" THEY REALISED THAT THINGS NEEDED TO CHANGE TO MAKE THEIR ACTIVITY MORE INCLUSIVE, SO THAT PEOPLE WHO WANTED TO TAKE PART NOW DIDN'T HAVE TO GO THROUGH WHAT THEY HAD TO. "**

WALK 1:

BORROWDALE TO SCAFELL PIKE

When you're ready for a hiking challenge, the Lake District must be your top destination. A full-day mountain ascent, Scafell Pike is the highest mountain in England and a bucket-list destination for hikers and outdoor enthusiasts around the world. It offers breathtaking views from its summit in the Lake District National Park of the surrounding landscapes and nearby Wastwater, the deepest lake in England.

Scafell Pike stands 978 metres (3,209 feet) above sea level and is an iconic part of the larger Scafell mountain range, which also includes Scafell and Great End. The summit can be accessed from various starting points, and there are several different routes, ranging in difficulty. The route here is one of the easiest and is suggested by www. scafellpike.org.uk. I highly recommend a thorough read of this site – it's a complete online guidebook to the area and full of important information about sensible preparation for a full-day mountain ascent.

Even given its challenging height and remoteness, you won't have the slopes to yourself – this is a very popular spot. Hiking to the top of Scafell Pike is an attractive challenge for many people, and according to the National Trust, 250,000 visitors a year try the ascent. There is no nearby public transport, and

Description: This is a mountainous route, and if you are an inexperienced hiker, consider doing it with a guide, a group or a more experienced companion

Distance: 14.5km (9 miles)/5.5 hours

Terrain: Rough rocky ground, grassy slopes, bog and occasional exposure

Toilets and refreshments: Public toilets at Wasdale. Pubs and tea rooms aplenty around Scafell Pike area

Getting there by public transport: 78 bus from Keswick to Seatoller (no closer public transport links), then carshare

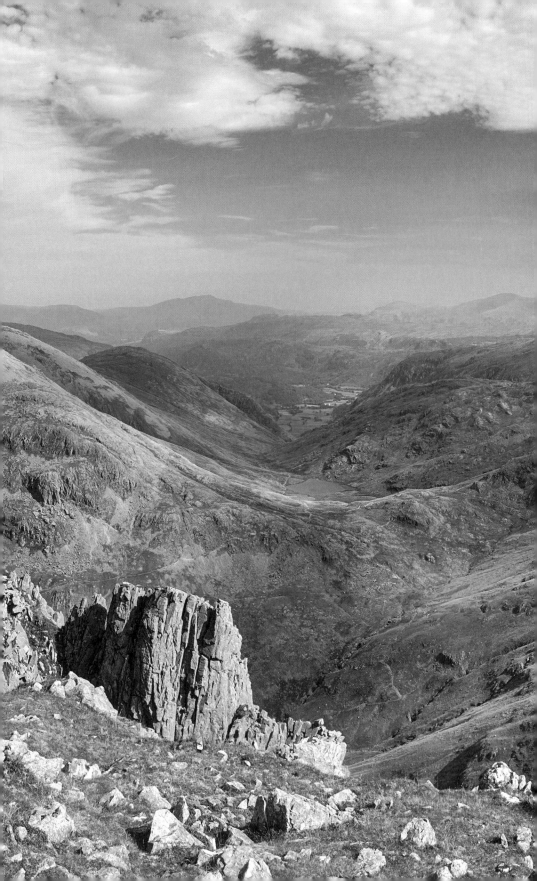

in peak times, the car park can become overcrowded, so the Trust encourages visitors to carshare.

Drive to the head of the Borrowdale valley and take the small left turn to Seathwaite. Park on the roadside (free of charge) at the end of the lane near Seathwaite Farm. This is usually very busy in summer and the farmer often opens up a field for extra paid parking.

Reaching Scafell Pike from Borrowdale is one of the most popular routes up Scafell Pike, and you'll soon see why. Set off along the track southwards through the lovely old farmyard and out into the open valley. Follow the track alongside the river to the delightful Stockley Bridge.

Cross the bridge and go through the gate, taking the path to the left, which continues to follow the river up Grains Gill. The path is well maintained; rising gradually at first, then more steeply alongside the tumbling waterfalls of Grains Gill until it meets a larger track running east–west beneath the towering cliffs of Great End directly in front of you.

Turn left (east) here and after 500 metres (547 yards), take the path that rises to the right up towards Esk Hause, where the stunning view south into Eskdale awaits. From Esk Hause, take the path westwards, climbing between Great End and Ill Crag, and across the boulder-strewn slopes of Broad Crag from where

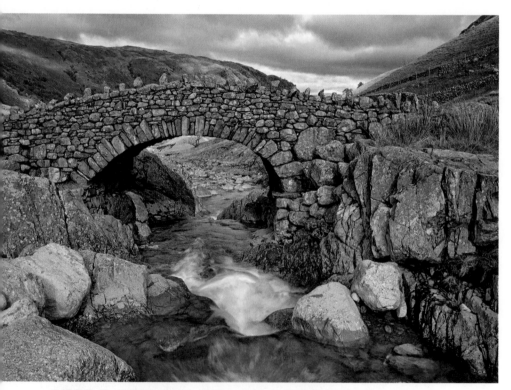

➡ ABOVE: The delightful Stockley Bridge. © Adobe Stock/Helen Hotson
➡ PAGE 127: the view from the top. © Adobe Stock/Nigel

FINDING YOUR FEET

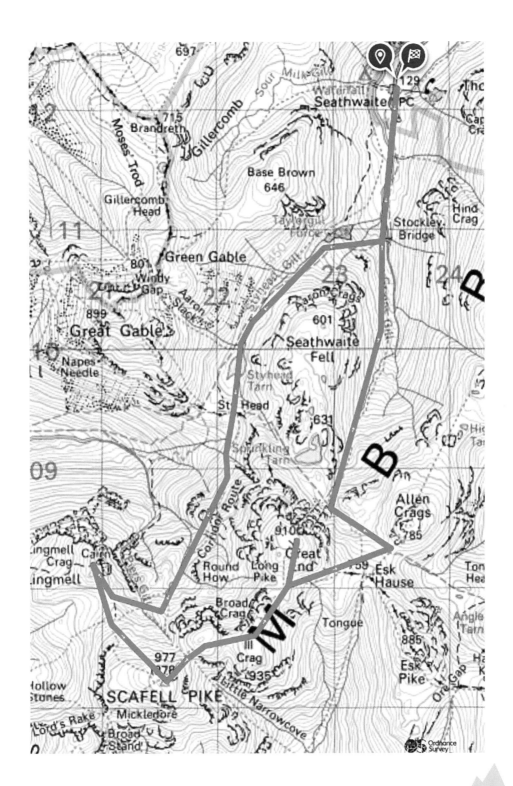

the towering summit of Scafell Pike finally comes into view.

Progress across the boulders here requires care and a twinge of disappointment awaits as you see the hard-earned height that must now be lost before the final ascent to the summit can begin! The final climb is steep and the ground is loose, but the summit plateau is soon reached and the giant cairn that marks the highest point in England comes back into view. It's time for a well-earned break to enjoy the sense of achievement and take in the breathtaking panoramic views.

But time waits for no (wo)man, and one of the most beautiful paths imaginable is still to come. From the summit, head north-west towards Lingmell. The path is a mass of boulders but well-marked with cairns and drops quickly down to Lingmell Col, where it meets the path rising up from Wasdale to the south-west. Here, take the path to the right (north-east), which is the beginning of the delightful 'Corridor Route'.

Contouring and dropping in stages, the path has towering peaks and crags to the right and dizzying views down into Wasdale to the left, until a short final climb leads up to Sty Head Pass.

Spend a few minutes sitting by Styhead Tarn looking back up towards Scafell Pike, as this will be your last view of the peak, before descending along the path to Styhead Gill until it reaches Stockley Bridge and the easy final stroll back to Seathwaite.

EXPERT ADVICE

Here is some advice from www.scafellpike.org.uk:

- Check the weather forecast and trail conditions before you start. Be prepared for changes in weather and visibility, even during the summer months.

- Wear comfortable hiking boots and dress in layers to accommodate temperature changes.

- Pack enough water, snacks and a packed lunch to keep your energy up.

- Carry a map and compass and consider using a GPS device or smartphone app for navigation.

- Start early in the day to ensure you have enough time to complete the hike and enjoy the experience.

- Be aware of your own fitness level and listen to your body. If the hike becomes too challenging, it's OK to turn back.

WALK 2:

GLENCOE

For all hikers, Scotland becomes an inevitable destination, offering as it does one of Europe's great wildernesses. The Glencoe Pass is a spectacular introduction. This trail forms part of the West Highland Way, Scotland's first long-distance route and its most popular. Beginning on the edge of Glasgow, it trails just over 150km (93 miles) to Fort William and the foot of Ben Nevis.

According to www.walkhighlands. co.uk, 'It offers tremendous variety, beginning in the pastoral landscapes beneath the Campsies, past the serene beauty of Loch Lomond, and on into increasingly rugged and majestic Highlands. It then crosses the vast, awe-inspiring expanse of Rannoch Moor, with a glimpse down Glencoe, before crossing the hills to lovely Loch Leven.

The route finally reaches Fort William via beautiful Glen Nevis.'

There's enough wilderness and poetry in those names for even the most committed English heart to yearn to journey north (and on a fast train, Glasgow is just four and a half hours from London, and from there, a National Express coach that stops in the village of Glencoe).

Glencoe was the site of a historic event, 'The Massacre of Glencoe', in 1692, and you will come across many references to the murder of the MacDonalds of Glencoe by Robert Campbell's troops. Some people think this tragic history adds to the grim grandeur of the landscape, which lent itself to cattle rustling between clans, or families.

Description: Challenging – steep and rough terrain

Distance: 6.4km (4 miles)/1.5–2 hours

Terrain: Rocky narrow ledges, requires climbing over boulders and crossing a river

Toilets and refreshments: Glencoe Visitor Centre and Glencoe Village for toilets and refreshments

Getting there by public transport: Train to Glasgow and Fort William, then a National Express coach from Fort William and Glasgow to Glencoe village

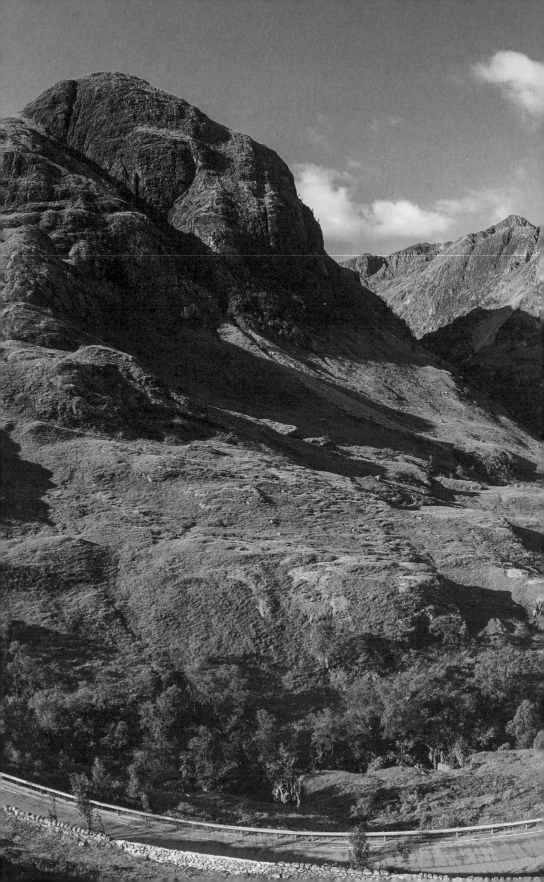

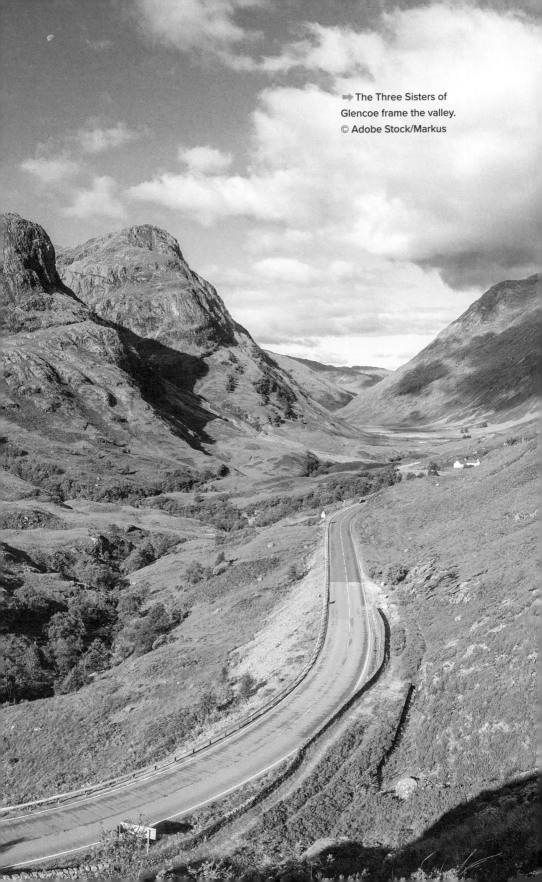

➡ The Three Sisters of Glencoe frame the valley.
© Adobe Stock/Markus

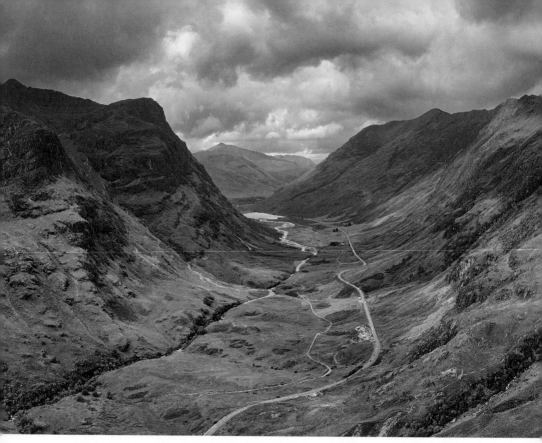

➡ **Looking down the valley.** © Adobe Stock/Markus Keller

Park in the large car park halfway up Glencoe. There is also a smaller car park a little further down the glen. Both get busy so try to arrive early in the day. There is a wonderful view of the glen from here — it is 16km (10 miles) long and less than 1km (0.6 miles) wide, so you will be surrounded by imposing mountains on all sides. There is also a fabulous view across to the Three Sisters — three peaks with impressive names: Beinn Fhada, Gearr Aonach and Aonach Dubh.

Follow the path downhill into the valley until you reach an old track through the glen; turn left before following the well-marked path off to the right towards the River Coe. This soon descends a wooden stairway to cross the River Coe (take care, these steps can get slippery) far below

in its gorge. Once across the bridge, the path becomes very rocky and rough and leads into a gorge between Beinn Fhada and Gearr Aonach. Again, be careful here (people have fallen into the gorge).

Scramble up the steep, rocky slope and continue on the path, which heads through woods and passes through a gate in the deer fence. Here, the path becomes a narrow ledge, with water flowing to your left. Look behind you for views of the Pass of Glencoe, a road that crosses Rannoch Moor, before entering the Glen.

Continue on the path, enjoying the tremendous rock walls on both sides. Watch out for the place where the path crosses the water on rough stepping stones. It is marked by two huge boulders. If there has been recent heavy

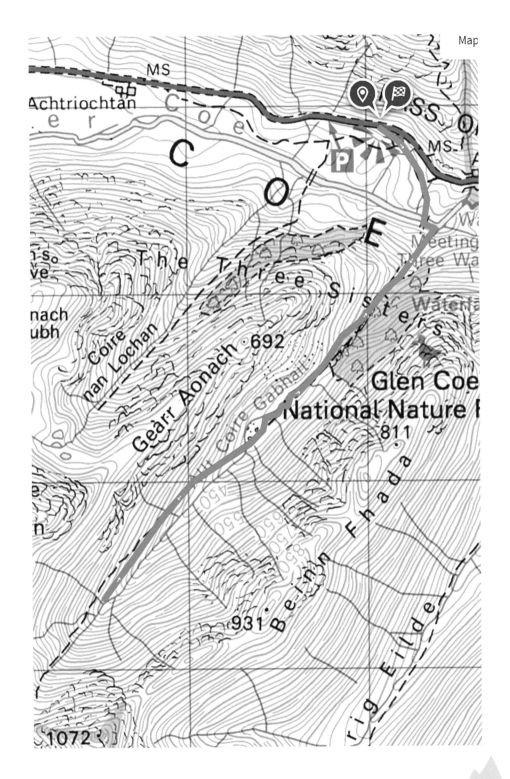

rain you might have to get your feet wet!

A short distance beyond here, the path scrambles up a rocky rake with a steep drop on the right. The scrambling is fairly straightforward, but it is steep, and might bring out a fear of heights in some hikers.

Once above here, the path has been improved with boulders placed to form steps, and there are more open views to Glencoe behind. After the roughest part of the hike, the path begins to descend into the Lost Valley. Until now totally obscured from view, this huge, flat area of stones and grass is completely cut off from Glencoe due to the rock falls in the gorge below.

It is worth exploring the flat area of the Lost Valley, which is littered with fallen rocks the size of houses, and admiring the great rock walls of Gearr Aonach and Beinn Fhada, which are so impressive.

Return to the car park via the same route.

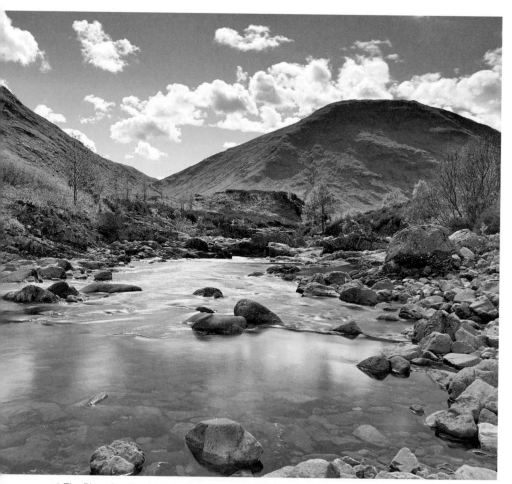

➡ The River Coe flows west along Glen Coe. © Adobe Stock/andreaskoch02

WALK 3:

LONDON WATERWAY HIKE: LIMEHOUSE BASIN TO LITTLE VENICE VIA THE GRAND UNION CANAL

The waterways of London are its lungs and its green heart. Skipping the crowded pavements and heading to the waterside gives Londoners a new way to enjoy their city, and visitors a free way to view countless architectural, cultural and natural wonders. With little free entertainment in our big cities generally, and London being particularly expensive, parents especially might appreciate something to do with the kids that doesn't leave them out of pocket at the end!

Routes that follow water are also excellent for beginners, or if you don't want to spend a lot of time wayfinding. If you're walking along a footpath that follows a river, a stretch of coastline or goes around a lake, it's really hard to

Description: Easy – surfaced paths, level or very gentle inclines

Distance: 14.5km (9 miles)/4 hours

Terrain: Urban, surfaced paths, occasional built-environment obstructions

Toilets and refreshments: Available at all points of the route

Getting there by public transport: Warwick Avenue tube station (ending at Limehouse DLR station)

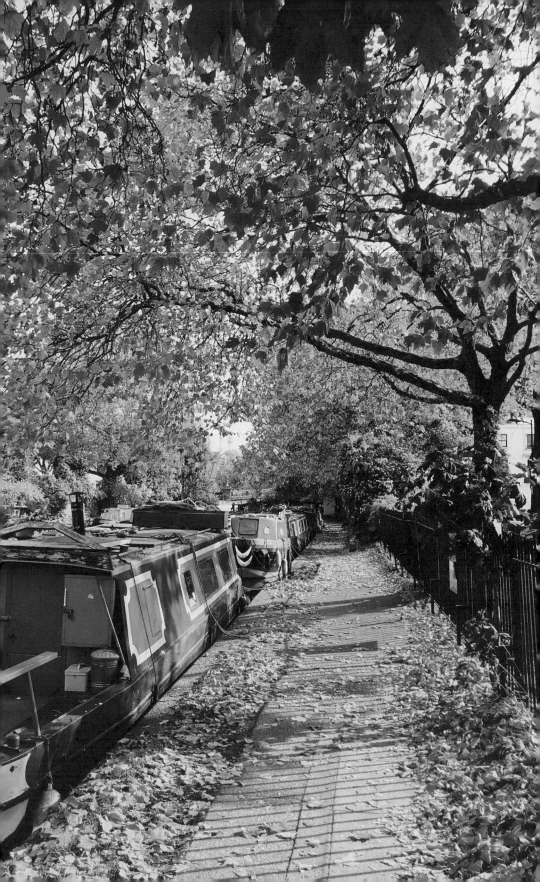

get lost! The Thames Path is the classic long-distance route, running 298km (185 miles) along the river from its source in the Cotswolds through several southern rural counties and into the urban heart of London. It's a life-long ambition for many hikers to complete the path, from its sleepy Cotswolds beginning to the end in Woolwich in East London, just a few miles from where the river flows into the sea.

For something a little different, the Regent's Canal provides a link from the River Thames at Limehouse Basin to the Grand Union Canal at Little Venice. Almost all of the walk can be done along the canal, and you will pass numerous live-aboard boats; the exotic animals of London Zoo peeking through the zoo's fences, which run along the canal path; as well as journeying through the ever-fashionable heart of Camden Town. This walk covers almost all of the 14.5km (9 miles) of the canal and shows you a completely different side of the capital – one that is green, laid-back and often very beautiful.

Begin your hike in Little Venice, a five-minute walk from Warwick Avenue tube station. Full of gorgeous Georgian buildings that back on to the canal, this is London as many people imagine it from films like *Notting Hill*. Consider a stop at Alfies Antique Market, where there are four floors of antiques to browse.

On the canal around here are many boats that people have adapted to live on full time. Especially in summer, these floating homes of the original boho Londoners are covered in flowers and pot plants and look really beautiful. Definitely one for the 'Gram! From here, follow the canal to Paddington Basin, where there has been a lot of leisure development, including cafes and shops,

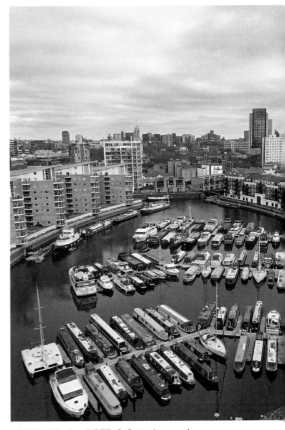

➡ Little Venice (LEFT: © Getty Images/ Alexander Spatari) and Limehouse Basin (ABOVE: © Adobe Stock/steve), in London.

to explore. You are about a five-minute walk from Paddington tube station here if you need a quick exit.

Next, the canal will lead you through Regent's Park, passing Lord's Cricket Ground and St John's Wood. In the park, but staying by the water, you'll soon encounter London Zoo. See how many animals you can spot from the towpath!

As Regent's Park turns into Camden, the houses become a grand assortment of old and new, and the vibe becomes more urban. Look out for Grand Union Walk, a row of silver pod-like houses built in the 1980s, and still futuristic-looking. Of course, Camden with its lock and market is a destination on its own – swerve off the towpath here for a drink, a wander around the market, or sample some of Camden's famous street food.

Soon, you'll come to King's Cross, recently regenerated and with the new destinations of Coal Drops Yard and Granary Square. New flats housed in old gasholders rise above the canal and there are lots of designer shops and food outlets.

For bookworms, a visit to Words on the Water is a must. It's a floating bookshop on a barge and you shouldn't miss it.

As you approach Islington, you will have a short detour on to the road at Angel where the towpath disappears, but you can swiftly rejoin it and enjoy the atmosphere of City Road Basin. Staying on the canal path, you can visit The Narrowboat pub, which is permanently on the water and a lovely place for a drink on a sunny day.

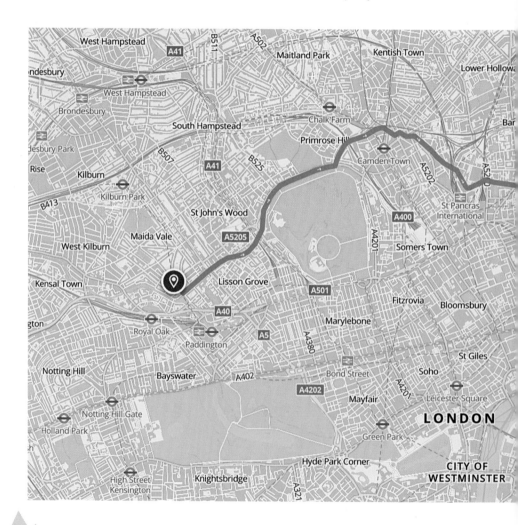

FINDING YOUR FEET

After Islington, you'll hike through Dalston, via the hipster village of Hoxton, and on to Victoria Park. This green space, one of London's biggest, will appear on your left. The park is a focus for the community: it is always busy, hosts festivals and has a cafe and art gallery. The canal splits at this point into the Hertford Union Canal, which leads towards Stratford and the Queen Elizabeth Olympic Park.

Take the arm that goes to Mile End Park. Consider popping up to the street to visit nearby Roman Road Market, an East End institution that has been going for over a century and a half and stretches for more than 800 metres (half a mile) through Bow.

Nearing the end of your hike, you'll come to Limehouse Basin, where the Thames meets Regent's Canal. The scene is a mix of watercraft, modern flats and buildings dating from the canal's opening in 1820. From here, it's a short walk to Limehouse DLR and the end of your journey.

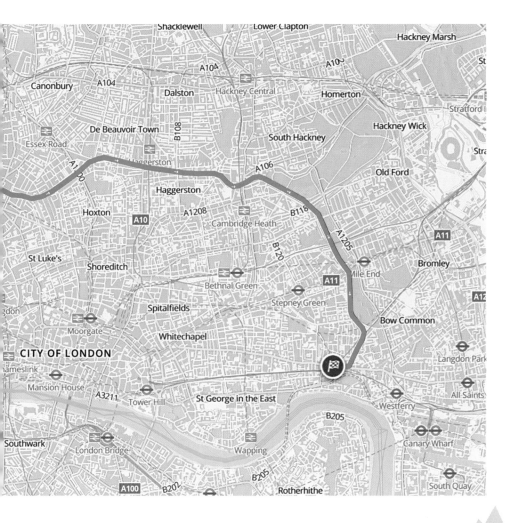

INTERVIEW: KWESIA _____

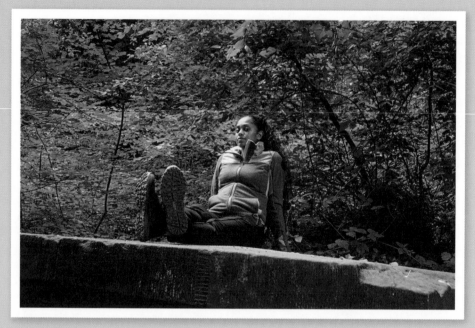

Photo © Kwesia

Kwesia: My name is Kwesia. I'm 24 and I live in South London. I'm the founder of City Girl in Nature, which is an initiative that connects the inner city with our natural world.

Rhiane: And how did you get into outdoor adventuring and what made you found City Girl in Nature?

Kwesia: So I first got into adventuring by going on an expedition in 2018 for three weeks with the British Exploring Society, and for me that was a life-changing experience. About two years later, I attended a conference run by Belinda Kirk called Adventure Mind. I saw that the space wasn't representing people like me, nor was it a space that I felt confident in. I felt like I could use my own experience to create a way to give back to the community.

Rhiane: What was the expedition that you did?

Kwesia: I went to the Peruvian Amazon for three weeks, where we went on hikes through the jungle, set up camp in different spaces and did

science projects. I was recording the whole time on a GoPro and there was a media person there called Emma who has worked with Planet Earth. So my first video was actually created from some of the videos that I captured on that expedition.

But for me, the element of not having a phone and being so far away from home with strangers who weren't from the same background as me, and being in nature, was really healing after a lot of the traumatic things I had faced. It was an opportunity for me to heal, essentially. I didn't see it like that while I was there, but afterwards, on reflection, I realised that's what had happened.

Rhiane: And how did you get chosen to go on the expedition with the British Exploring Society?

Kwesia: I was working in a youth club called Caius House in Clapham Junction, with a project that I used to do work with called Black Minds Matter UK. It was giving young people kind of the opportunity to have alternative therapies, like music therapy, yoga and art therapy. A guy from the British Exploring Society came and presented this opportunity and no one was really interested. I was the only one who was into it, I suppose, and the person who ran the youth club got funding to help me to go on the expedition. I was fortunate to get a sponsor.

> ## 66
> ## PUSH THE BOUNDARIES. BURST YOUR OWN BUBBLE. THERE ARE SO MANY GEMS TO BE FOUND OUTSIDE YOUR COMFORT ZONE.
> ## 99

Rhiane: What exactly does City Girl in Nature do? What kind of activities? You have a web series don't you?

Kwesia: I have an online series, that's where I started. I felt that medium was the best way that I could kind of show what I represent. I got people that I found inspirational, including yourself, and interviewed them. I used music and incorporated visuals as well, showing what trainers people are wearing. That's all part of showing where I'm coming from and making it relatable to the young people whom I'm trying to reach. A few people were within the outdoors industry. Off the back of that, I started being noticed in the outdoors world, and I started connecting with more people. I started getting opportunities within that, but at the same time I started giving grassroots workshops. Going into schools, for instance, and speaking at certain conferences that were not necessarily places where people like you and me would be. I was using that as a platform to try to change the narrative within the outdoors industry, not just on their part but in our world too. Bridging the gap between the two.

Rhiane: So now you're influencing policy and you're going into these spaces. How would you sum up the new perspective you bring to the space?

Kwesia: I feel like I bring my authentic self. I guess one thing about me is that I never change. I always speak from where I'm coming from. Being an inner-city girl, coming from the endz. I like being able to show and be myself in this space, despite it not being representative. I want to be able to make nature cool.

> **"**
>
> ## I LIKE BEING ABLE TO SHOW AND BE MYSELF IN THIS SPACE, DESPITE IT NOT BEING REPRESENTATIVE. I WANT TO BE ABLE TO MAKE NATURE COOL.
>
> **"**

Rhiane: So you're saying that you're not doing that code-switching thing with them, and you're just showing up as your authentic, unapologetic self. You're showing up as *you*.

Kwesia: I feel that the work that I do is not just about trying to get people involved with what *I'm* doing. It's also about allowing people to see that it's a tool that *they* can use, that nature could play a part in their lives more generally.

Rhiane: Being authentic is obviously what draws people towards you. And I like that you're trying to show people that nature is a tool and that everybody can use it at some point in their lives. What was the response like to your series?

Kwesia: It was really impactful because people were like, what? Who *is* this? What's she doing? It was just different, like a glitch in the matrix, set against where I'm from and my story. The most satisfying thing for me is that people I'm working with see the direct impact on them. Even family and friends are wanting to be involved. Working with grassroots community groups and going into schools, when young people ask questions, that's the best kind of impact. People get a new perspective through my experience. Does that make sense?

Rhiane: It does, definitely. It's all about being relatable, isn't it? And obviously, you're very relatable to the people who are in your community – that's how you engage them. You mentioned before that you found being in the outdoors healing. Would you say that that's the main kind of benefit you've noticed in your life since you started doing this?

Kwesia: I'd say the core thing is the healing element of it, and how it's good to use it as a tool to nourish my mental and physical well-being. Even my spiritual well-being – kind of aligning myself. I like using myself as an example, but I don't necessarily tell people how they should do it. You can only lead by example.

Rhiane: I notice that you recently won an award. Congratulations!

Kwesia: Thanks. It was the 2023 John Spedan Lewis Emerging Leader Award. It is given to people making an impact, and for me it's for my impact on the natural world. It's just for the work that I've done with my series. Getting an award motivated me but really, it's always about my community.

Rhiane: What advice would you give to somebody who is looking to find their feet in the outdoors? Do you have any takeaways?

Kwesia: I think it always comes down to experience. I'd say, try to experience things. There are so many gems to find outside of your comfort zone, even if you might feel like it's not for you or you don't see yourself doing it. Just give things a try. Push the boundaries. Burst your own bubble.

INTERVIEW: CHANTELLE LINDSAY

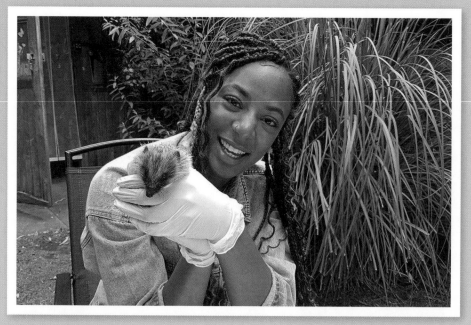

Photos © Chantelle Lindsay

Chantelle: I'm Chantelle Lindsay. I'm 29 and I live on the borders of Croydon, South London. I am the Nature in Mind coordinator for the London Wildlife Trust, a youth programme based around mental health and nature. I'm also a TV presenter.

Rhiane: What do you present at the moment?

Chantelle: I have a show called *Teeny Tiny Creatures with Chantelle and Rory* – no idea if it's going to be recommissioned! It's about getting young people excited about the littler creatures. I also do some work on *Springwatch* and other nature shows.

Rhiane: And you do voice-over work now as well?

Chantelle: Yes, I do things about climate change at the moment, but hopefully I'll be a voice-over artist one day.

Rhiane: And how did you start taking an interest in nature?

Chantelle: I just feel like I've always loved wildlife. When I was little, I tried to adopt other people's pets because I couldn't have my own. I always found nature really peaceful and awe-inspiring. I first thought, *I'm going to be a vet!* because that was the only role I knew of in the wildlife sector. Then I thought, *No, I don't want to do that – it's too many years in school.* And I just couldn't put anything to sleep – I'd be a wreck!

Rhiane: Did you go out with your family into nature?

Chantelle: Yes, my mum always tried her best to get us out and about. I always remember her taking us to the Natural History Museum and bike riding and into the woods and stuff like that. But I'm the wildlife nutter in my house. My sisters and my mum have different connections with it, like my mum loves gardening. She's very much a person of the earth.

Rhiane: How many years have you been working professionally in the field?

Chantelle: Four years now. I started with the London Wildlife Trust in 2019 on the Keep it Wild traineeship. I quit my job working for a pensions call centre, which was crippling my soul. I had come back from Spain where I was teaching English, and the only reason I came back to England was to find a job in wildlife conservation – it took me two years. I saw the traineeship and thought, *Oh my God, it's paid!* It had an emphasis on getting young people and people from marginalised communities into the sector.

Rhiane: So, you've come through one of the London Wildlife Trust's programmes. What would you say makes people resonate with you as a person?

Chantelle: Well, my passion for nature shines through. I've got a degree in animal behaviour but it wasn't very academic, so I don't know all the Latin names and all the jargon, but that's relatable for people. I think my journey is as well. I think a lot of Black people struggle to get into this sector. It's a real privilege to be able to follow your passion.

Rhiane: Have you noticed any kind of shifts in the sector, positive ones that are genuine and meaningful?

Chantelle: I'm in a bit of a bubble at the London Wildlife Trust. In the countryside, it would be a completely different experience. But a lot of organisations now are rolling out traineeships that are paid, so people are investing in young people, not expecting them to work for free as much as they used to. And I think for our communities, that's meaningful because we can't afford to just give up all our time for free.

Rhiane: How do you feel when people say you're a role model? Does it feel like a pressure, or does it make you feel proud?

Chantelle: It makes me feel really proud! The last couple of years were tough, with my presenting career taking off, I felt like I was going at 100 miles an hour. But when people approach you, it's just amazing. A woman came up to me and said, 'It's just amazing seeing you on television.' And then there were the wonderful messages I got after my first ever *Springwatch* appearance. There were so many from Black women, who said, 'It's so nice to see another woman of colour on the show.' Sometimes I feel I'm not doing enough to open the doors to people behind me, but then I have to stop myself and think, *Calm down! Get yourself right first!*

Rhiane: You're an idol for little kids as well. Do you get recognised by them?

Chantelle: It's more the parents than the kids!

Rhiane: Do you see yourself going into the media full time?

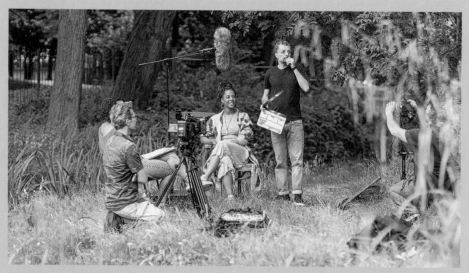

➡ Nature is my passion.

Chantelle: I've always wanted to be a wildlife conservationist. So much of my identity is about being on the ground, getting my hands dirty, doing practical stuff. The ideal would be to travel the world and film different projects.

Rhiane: You need to pitch that to somebody!

Chantelle: I'm thinking about it. But progress in terms of representation is so slow in TV. I've worked with an Asian filmmaker. I've worked with a Black videographer. It's not like we're not there or we're invisible, it's just people are so lazy in this industry and nepotism perpetuates the gatekeeping. So now I'm thinking, *How can I do this on my own?*

Rhiane: You should start off with a YouTube series, then build it from there. What advice would you give to somebody who was looking to find their way, not just in the outdoors, or who wants to try something new?

Chantelle: Go for it and try not to have imposter syndrome. It's natural, but it helps you to realise what you bring to the table. I think a lot of the time we go into a space and we start shrinking ourselves and feeling like we're inadequate. But the reason you're there in the first place is because you've got something to bring.

When I first started at the London Wildlife Trust, I was working with so many amazing people, but I was so daunted, thinking, *I don't know anything so I shouldn't say anything*, and I'd start to doubt why I was there. I think that has an extra layer on it for Black women as well. I wondered, *Are they just trying to tick a box?* It really played on my insecurities and left me questioning if I was worthy.

Also, try not to be intimidated. And focus on what your speciality is, because with social media, everything is so saturated. It feels like you're never going to break the mould. Just bring your life, just bring you. That's all you can do. Allow that to shine and lead with that.

66

IMPOSTER SYNDROME IS NATURAL. IT HELPS YOU REALISE WHAT YOU BRING TO THE TABLE.

99

WALK 4:

MANNINGTREE TO DEDHAM VALE

This hike is through an Area of Outstanding Natural Beauty that straddles the counties of Essex and Suffolk. It has some truly stunning scenery of chocolate-box perfection and is a great destination at any time of the year. In summer, the countryside is lusciously verdant and alive with insects going about their business. In winter, the leafless trees and rolling mists give the whole area a mysterious atmosphere, and because the trees are leafless, you can really appreciate the wonderful views over Dedham Vale.

This was the birthplace of the famous landscape painter John Constable, and if it seems a little familiar, it's because his images have become synonymous with this part of the world. You might even recognise some scenes from his widely

Description: Easy, on generally flat grass and gravel paths with some moderate slopes

Distance: 6.4km (4 miles)/1.5 hours return from Manningtree to Flatford. Optional loop to Dedham adds another 4.8km (3 miles)/1 hour

Terrain: Can be muddy after wet weather – take care when walking on riverside sections of the route

Toilets and refreshments: WC at Manningtree Station, Flatford and Dedham villages. National Trust riverside tearoom and shop at Flatford; other shops and pubs at Dedham

Getting there by public transport: Manningtree Station (London Liverpool Street to Ipswich line)/services to Manningtree Station and Dedham from Colchester and Ipswich. The Painter's Trail cycle route passes through the Stour Valley to Manningtree Station

reproduced paintings; *The Hay Wain* and *Boat-Building Near Flatford Mill*, for example, were painted close to this route. Flatford Bridge Cottage hosts an exhibition on Constable. There are loads of gorgeous photo opportunities, as well as wildlife to spot, including kingfishers, otters, woodpeckers and barn owls.

Leave Manningtree Station exit and descend the ramp to the right. The footpath starts from the end of the ramp in the car park. After leaving the car park, turn right along a track, then right again under a railway bridge. Follow the path

across the meadows until you reach the river. This is the Stour.

Turn left and follow the riverside path, through the Cattawade Marshes. (Do not wander off the path into the marshes. They are criss-crossed with streams and wildlife hiding in the reeds. These are best observed with binoculars.)

After another 1.6km (1 mile) or so, you will see an old flood defence barrier but don't cross it. Follow the path on the bank to the hamlet of Flatford. As the path nears Flatford Lock you can see the large house and watermill owned by the

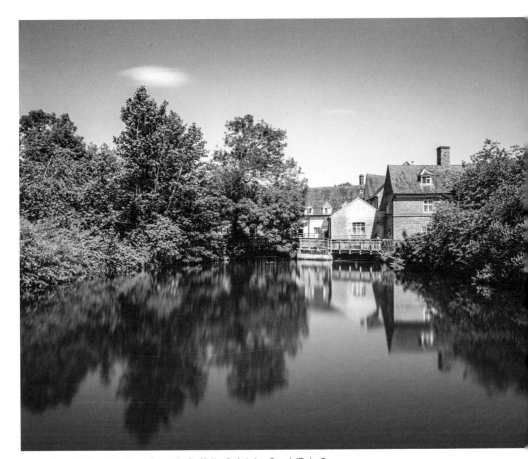

➡ Flatford Mill on the River Stour in Suffolk. © Adobe Stock/Fela Sanu

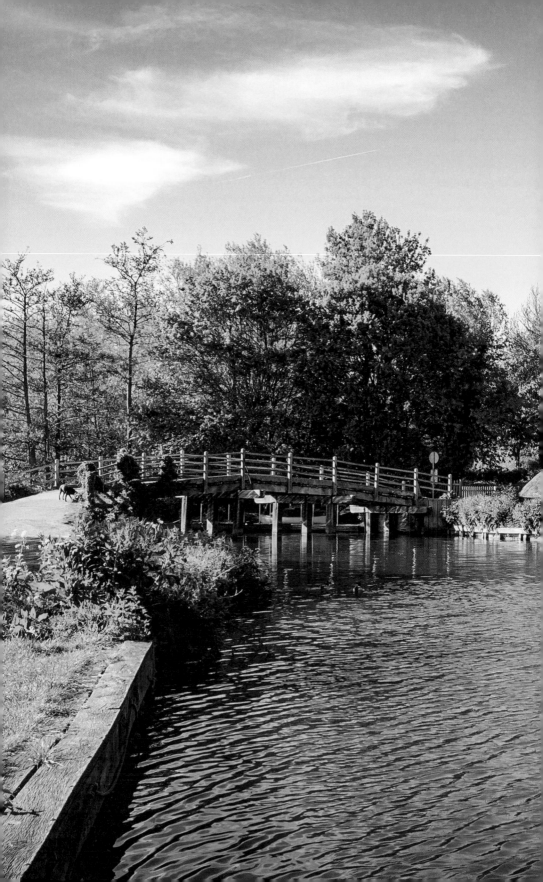

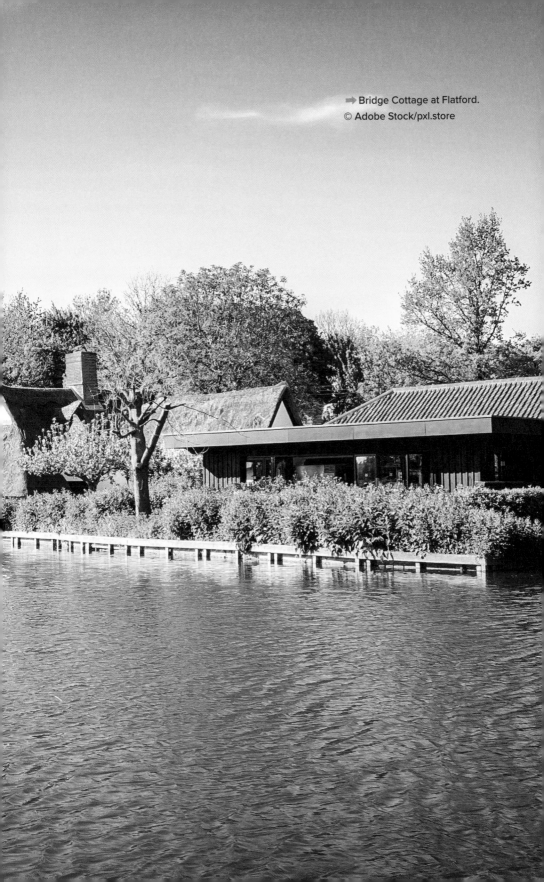

artist John Constable's father. From here, you are very close to Flatford Mill and Willy Lott's House, which are kept just as they looked in Constable's day by the National Trust.

Pass the lock and walk across Flatford Bridge to reach the lovely thatched Bridge Cottage. Here, there's a tearoom and a Constable exhibition. Turn left at the top of the lane and after 100 metres (110 yards), take the footpath running parallel to the road. Panoramic views over the vale can be had from the top of the hill. Turn left into Fen Lane.

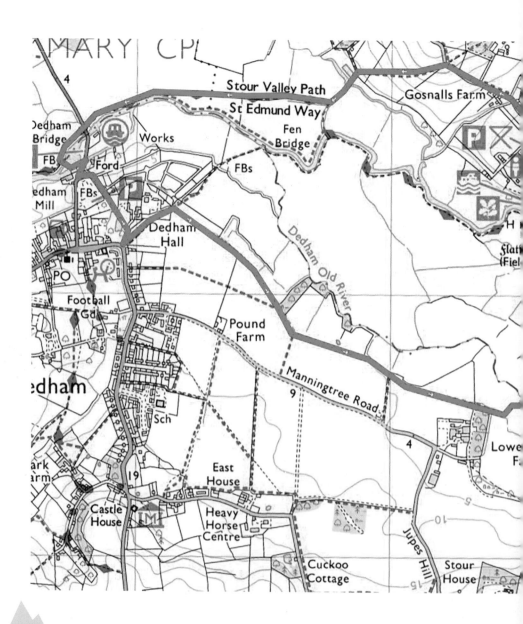

Shortly after crossing a bridge, turn right along a tree-lined footpath. Cross riverside meadows, until you reach a bridge at Dedham. Leave the village on a footpath after the drive to Dedham Hall. Follow this to Flatford, bearing left at the National Trust sign to Dedham Hall Farm.

The river leads back to Bridge Cottage across water meadows. From Bridge Cottage, retrace your steps, via Flatford Bridge and Cattawade Marshes to return to Manningtree.

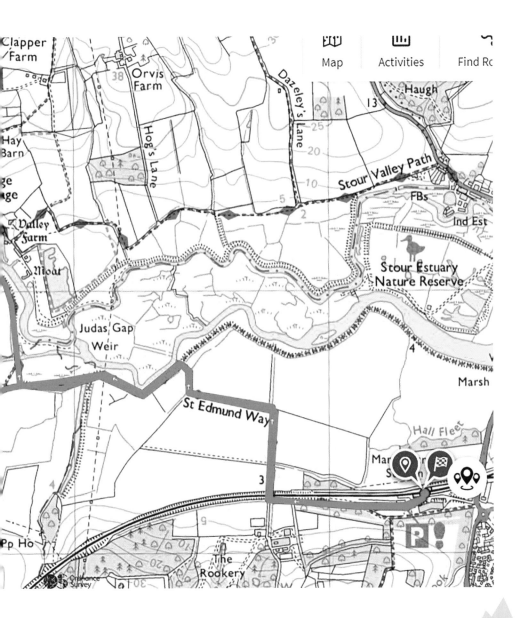

WALK 5:

OUSE VALLEY

The River Ouse flows through the heart of Sussex and out to the English Channel at Newhaven. This route closely follows the Egrets Way project to link Lewes and Newhaven. Some of it is still under construction, and more information can be found at www.egretsway.org.uk.

The Egrets Way runs north to south, crossing the South Downs Way at Southease. This is where you start your walk. Southease railway station is so small it is not even on a proper street – you will exit on to a single-track road and encounter a sign immediately outside the station that points to both the South Downs Way and the youth hostel – YHA South Downs, which is around 180 metres (200 yards) away, has reasonable accommodation and an excellent licensed cafe. However, ignore both these options and head towards Southease Bridge, an aged metal and wood crossing over the Ouse. The bridge takes you over the river and on to the other side. You can drop down straight on to the riverside footpath, which wends high above the tidal waters flowing below in the valley.

Please note: the River Ouse is tidal. When the tide is out, the river appears to be very low in its channel, but the tide brings with it very strong currents, so going into the water can mean being pulled down into the sea or getting stuck in the mud. Exercise caution.

The walk follows the river, which snakes through agricultural land and offers views up to the hills of the South Downs and south towards Newhaven.

Description: A beginner's hike, with very little on-road walking and marvellous views

Distance: 6.4km (4 miles)/1.5 hours

Terrain: Lanes, tracks (some muddy and narrow), gentle hills

Toilets and refreshments: YHA South Downs has a great cafe, or there are plenty of pubs and cafes in Newhaven

Getting there by public transport: Train from Brighton or Lewes to Southease; then Newhaven Town to Lewes and Brighton

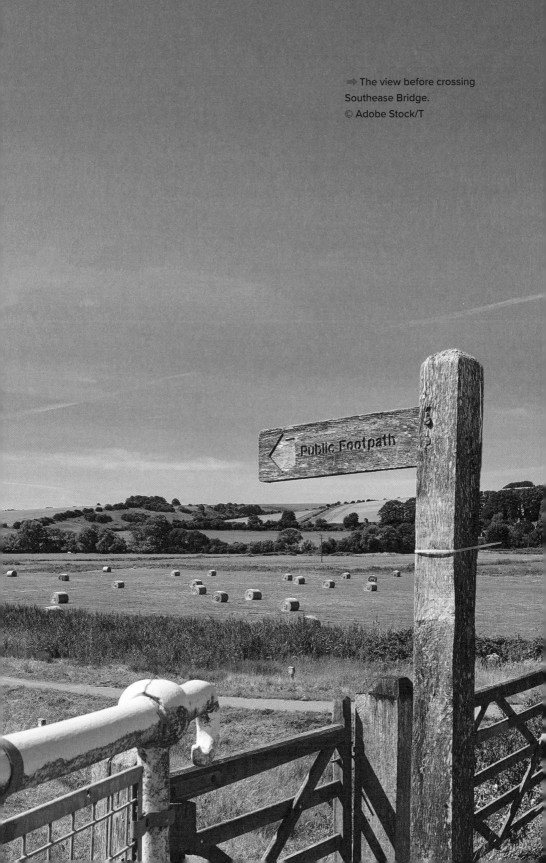

Public Footpath

Follow the riverside path until Deans Farm, where you will find the path peters out into inaccessible private land.

Here, follow the roadway south, bearing left off the riverside path, until you see a pair of ornate double wrought-iron gates on your right. There is a narrow access point to the left of the gate. Pass through this and take the track that runs parallel to the tarmac driveway (it is marked on the map as a public bridleway). Continue to follow this path as it climbs up the hill in front of you. It will become narrow and perhaps muddy, but as you climb and take the path around the brow of the hill, fantastic views of the river valley beneath you will be revealed.

Continue to follow this path over the brow of the hill and down through fields into the picturesque village of Piddinghoe with its ancient church and wisteria-covered cottages. From here, you will find the path directs you towards the riverside once again. If you look back, you will see a small quay on the riverside with a number of boats, a reminder of the

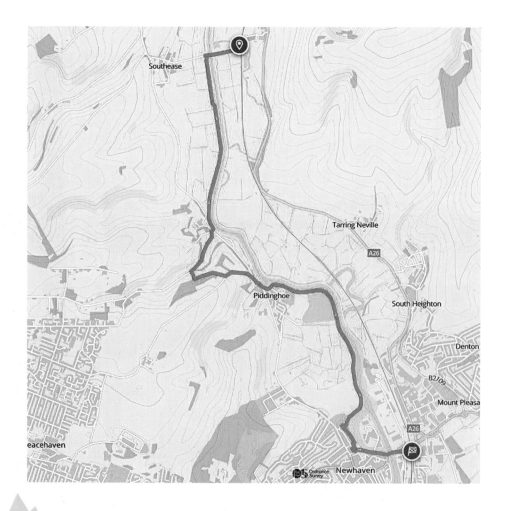

FINDING YOUR FEET

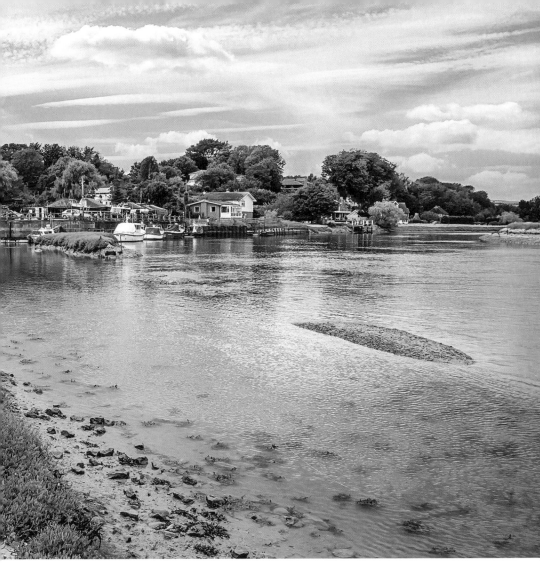

⇒ Looking towards Piddinghoe village from the River Ouse. © Adobe Stock/Nicola

time when Piddinghoe village was at the centre of smuggling goods inland using the Ouse waterway to avoid taxes.

Once back on the riverside, you will soon see Newhaven and its industrial port (and impressive futuristic warehouse) in front of you. Beyond it you will see the bridge that crosses the Ouse and gives access to Newhaven Town train station.

Follow the riverbank past the industrial port and keep going as domestic fishing and pleasure vessels take over. There are fascinating houseboats to look at before you eventually come to the main road that leads to Newhaven Bridge (NB this is a swing bridge and sometimes closes for tall boats).

Once you hit the main road, use the pedestrian walkway to cross the bridge (as the only crossing point, it is usually busy with road traffic here). From here, you can follow the pedestrian signs for Newhaven Town Station, which is next to the town's ferry terminal.

INTERVIEW: SORAYA ABDEL—HADI ____

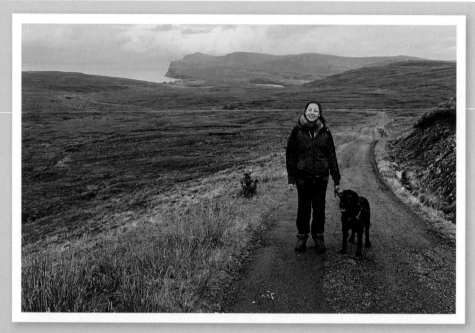

Photos © Soraya Abdel-Hadi

Soraya: My name is Soraya Abdel-Hadi. I am 37 and I'm the founder and director of All The Elements. I am also an award-winning writer, artist, sustainability professional and coach. I live in Hampshire.

Rhiane: And what is All The Elements?

Soraya: It's a non-profit network for everyone creating change around diversity in the UK outdoors.

Rhiane: Why did you start it?

Soraya: I was a writer originally, and then I moved into sustainability as my career. But I continued writing and one of the things I was writing about was diversity in the outdoors. And when I did my dissertation on authentic leadership for women, I realised that I wasn't stepping up into that space myself. I wasn't 'walking the walk', so I decided to start putting myself out there. But I realised that this work is really hard!
    And, though I could see people on social media doing like epic things, there wasn't a central space where I could see everybody. I felt like I

needed a network. Then I reached out to a few people, including yourself, about the fact that I was thinking of setting one up. And most people said that it would be really great to be able to talk to other people who also work in the space.

I'm really passionate about it being intersectional, including all diversities, so that people can peer-to-peer learn across those areas. It makes the community bigger, more interesting and more exciting.

Rhiane: And how did you get into outdoor adventure. Were your family outdoorsy?

Soraya: I am mixed race – my mum is white British and my dad is Black Sudanese and I was raised here in the UK. My mum's family are super outdoorsy and I grew up playing in the woods with my cousins and my brother, walking their dog and going to beach picnics. All of that was really normal in my life. I was also horse obsessed from when I was tiny and where I lived was suburbia, but semi-rural. When I was a teenager, I was lucky enough to get my own horse and I had a part-time job to contribute towards paying for him. He meant I was outdoors all the time, because once you have a horse, unless you are super-rich and somebody else looks after them for you, all of your time is spent riding or in muddy fields.

Rhiane: As you built the network, what made you think, *Yes, this is it! All The Elements is really necessary, I'm really going to stick with this*?

66
WE ONLY HAVE ONE LIFE, SO JUST JUMP.
99

Soraya: We've run socials online since the very beginning, and they've continued to be super popular. People meet and they go off and do projects together and I hear about it a year later! Since then I've done over 350 individual one-on-one calls with people working in the space to talk through what they're working on and what they're interested in, what they need, and who they might want to connect with. In this space, as you know, people are asking you for stuff all the time. But the community is amazing. That's the thing, that's why I keep doing it – because they're incredible.

Rhiane: When we get emails that say, 'Can you do this, this, this and this?', I reply, 'Oh you should just contact All The Elements!'

Soraya: But that's exactly what we're there for! The whole point of us is to take the pressure off, we're the support, at the centre of the community. If I didn't get paid, if all the brands didn't want to work with us any more, I would still run the community because that's the most important bit.

Rhiane: What would you say is the biggest issue that people come to you with?

Soraya: That's a great question. It's been a really interesting process because so many groups set up during Covid-19. So originally, we had loads of people asking if they should be a CIC, for example. Then I had a period where people were asking about kit. Too many people were setting up kit libraries, and that's a conversation that is still ongoing. I feel like they should all be talking to each other so that we don't end up with 150 tiny kit libraries!
     Training was a big one at the beginning as well. Should our outdoor instructors be trained? And now I feel like it's more, how do we write an effective EDI [equality, diversity and inclusion] policy? How do we scale up? Or how do we choose the right opportunities? How much should I charge if someone's asking me to do a talk? I get asked a lot about whether big organisations are racist. I'm like, I don't know!

Rhiane: What would you say is your biggest challenge in terms of running the organisation, apart from funding and capacity?

Soraya: I find my biggest challenge is that I am representing everyone. When I go somewhere repping All The Elements, it's 300 people and 300 people's opinions and 300 people's approaches, and that's tricky. It's even trickier, because for some reason people who *don't* work in this space, but who might want to work with our members, think we're all the same. Trying to explain to them that there's isn't one answer to their question, and there isn't a singular way that a group is going to react if they approach them – well, that's really tough.

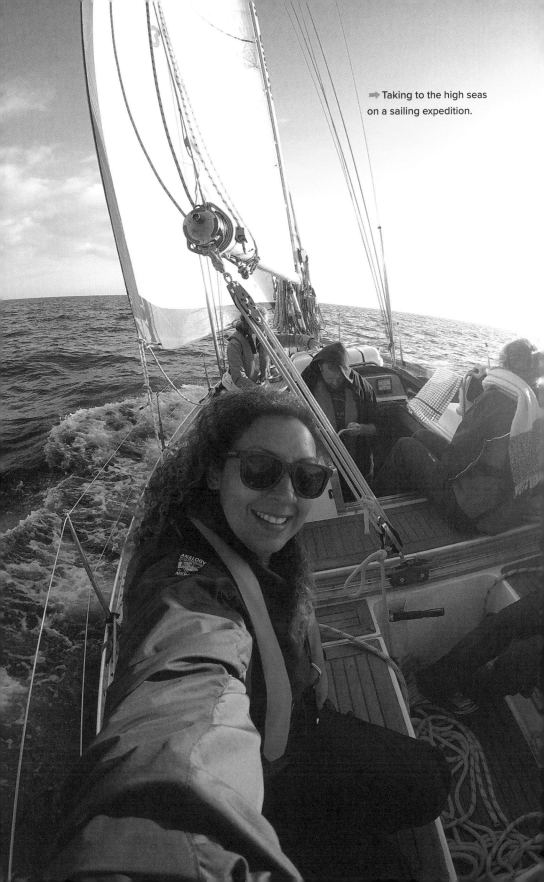

Taking to the high seas on a sailing expedition.

Also, and this is a very honest answer, I'm currently looking at how I can I have pretty strong opinions and continue to do this work. I have an activist background, and this year, I've realised that I need to find a way to continue to do my own thing, without it impacting on the organisation, which has to represent so many different people with their own, completely valid, lived experiences.

Rhiane: You only ever get invited to talk about one thing! You're not allowed to be an individual with your own interests, which I find really jarring.

Soraya: Yeah, that's totally it.

Rhiane: So you said you did horse riding when you were younger. But I also know that you were a climbing instructor, weren't you?

Soraya: So my career has been super wiggly! Before I retrained in sustainability, I worked at an equestrian magazine for four years, and it was an amazing job, but the pay was like awful. When I went back to uni to retrain, I took up climbing and I love it. It gets you into your body and makes you really feel in the moment – it switches your brain off. All you can think about is how to get the next move. I'm also a bit scared of heights, so it gives me a buzz. I became a part-time instructor because I loved it so much.

After university, I booked to go on a trip to canoe down the Mississippi River with a bunch of strangers. It's the best experience I think I've ever had, so strange and so weird. We were in open Canadian canoes, and we also paddleboarded. Paddleboarding on the Mississippi is really easy if you're going downstream, but less easy if you need to get across to a bank because it travels so quickly. We were camping on sandbanks and that's when I started painting, too.

One of the people organising that trip was an ocean advocate called Emily Penn, and she had just started an organisation called X Expedition – sailing expeditions looking at plastics and toxins in the ocean all over the world. I volunteered for her, and we organised around-Britain expeditions, stopping in I think five different ports. Eventually I got to go sailing myself, from Vancouver to Seattle via the Broken Group Islands.

Rhiane: Oh, that sounds great.

Soraya: It was really good. It was so exciting. The Broken Group Islands were incredibly beautiful and we got to meet with local First Nations communities to talk about the importance of the islands in their history and moving forwards. And then on the last day we finally saw orcas and I was emotional, the way they were moving through the water. I thought, *I can't believe people put them in tanks. Why would you do that?*

Rhiane: It's really overwhelming when you see certain things in nature. Last week I saw my first seal up in North Yorkshire. You've come so far now, what are the challenges you face as a community leader would you say?

Soraya: Beyond all the basic things of funding and capacity, I think being the face of something has taken me a long time to grow into and I would still prefer that people understood that it's community led and community run. When people try to give me credit for All The Elements, what people don't understand is that it's about the community — without the community, there's nothing.

Also, when I first started, because I do come from a pretty privileged background, I felt very uncomfortable speaking on behalf of other people. It was why I hadn't worked in diversity before because people would ask me all the time, 'How do we get more people *like you* here?' And I would reply, 'What, from Hampshire?' I always felt like, who am I to speak on behalf of all people of colour? Especially because I haven't faced a lot of struggles. So, at the beginning, that was probably the hardest thing, stepping into that role.

Rhiane: If you were going to give advice to someone who was looking to find their feet in the outdoors or in any other element of life, what would you say?

Soraya: Be brave. It's going to be fine. It might seem scary and it's hard, but we only have one life, so just jump. What's the worst thing that's going to happen? You don't go surfing again? Or you decide mountains aren't your thing? Just try things. Don't be scared to be crap at them. It's not about being good at things. It's about having those experiences.

66
IT'S NOT ABOUT BEING GOOD AT THINGS. IT'S ABOUT HAVING THOSE EXPERIENCES.
99

WALK 6:

PORT EYNON TO RHOSSILI

This is a sometimes beautiful, challenging, hilly route along the cliffs and beaches of the Wales Coastal Path. It is located in the Gower Peninsula, one of the first places in Britain to be named an Area of Outstanding Natural Beauty. With cliffs and woodlands ringed by sparkling beaches, the Gower peninsula is justly popular with hikers, but its abundant wildlife also lures birdwatchers and the stunning beaches attract surfers and holidaymakers.

This walk includes spectacular coastal scenery, including the iconic Worm's Head, a narrow cliff that juts out into the sea and is only accessible around low tide (so do check tide times before you set out!). Rhossili is one of Britain's most wonderful beaches: this walk really is a treat for the senses.

If you get off the bus from Swansea in Port Eynon you need first to walk to the seafront and head for the western end of the beach, where there is a path next to the youth hostel. This trail leads to the Wales Coast Path, and you will follow it all the way.

Follow the path up the cliff, where you will see a commemorative standing stone on the summit.

Here, you will find a grass path along the cliff top that drops down to a gate and down to Overton Mere. Continue on this undulating path over Overton Cliff,

Description: Moderate to hard with steep sections, but navigation is easy

Distance: 11.3km (7 miles)/2.5 hours

Terrain: Grassy paths, with possible stones and rocks. Muddy in winter

Toilets and refreshments: Cafes and facilities at Port Eynon and Rhossili

Getting there by public transport: Nearest train station is Swansea. From there, bus to Port Eynon

with the Bristol Channel crashing against dramatic cliffs on your left.

After a while, the path divides, with the official Wales Coast Path going to the right to a point higher on the cliff slightly inland and through a field. On your left, an alternative but more challenging path skirts the cliffs and rewards you with amazing scenery. However, after about 1km (0.6 miles), at Long Hole Cave, the

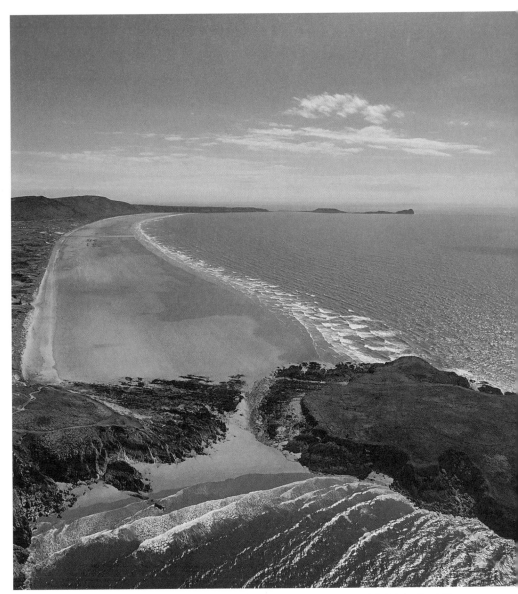

➡ ABOVE: The magnificent curve of Rhossili Bay looking towards Worms Head. © Adobe Stock/Terry
➡ OVERLEAF: Worms Head at the end of the Gower Peninsula. © Adobe Stock/Stephen Davies

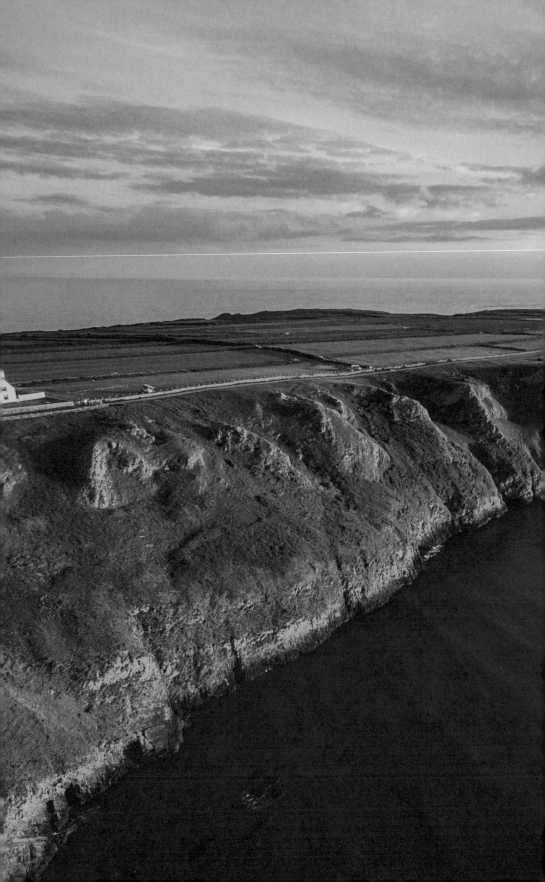

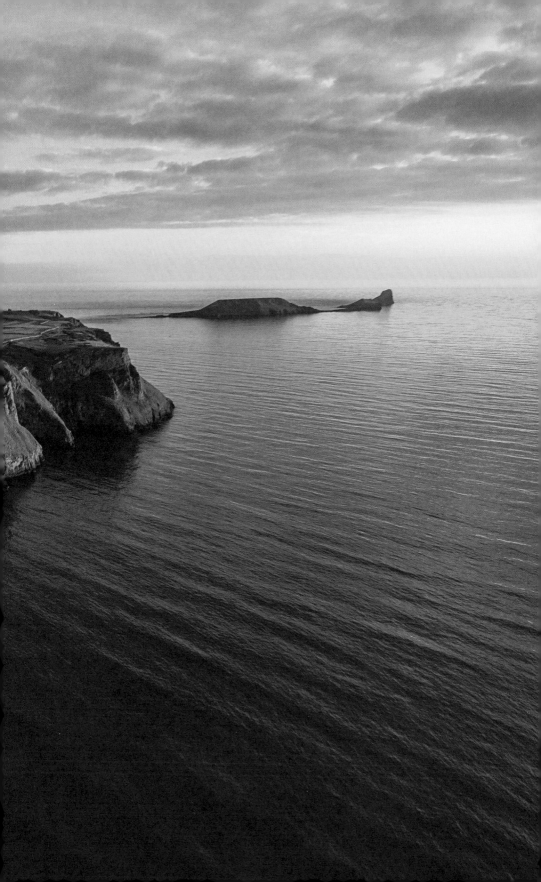

lower path is closed, and you will need to head back up to the cliff top to take the official path. This continues past pretty Mewslade Bay, where there is a steep drop down to the small valley before a steep ascent back up again.

Next, the path will take you past Fall Bay beach and you will begin to see the Worm's Head, an iconic rocky outcrop emerging like a dragon rising from the

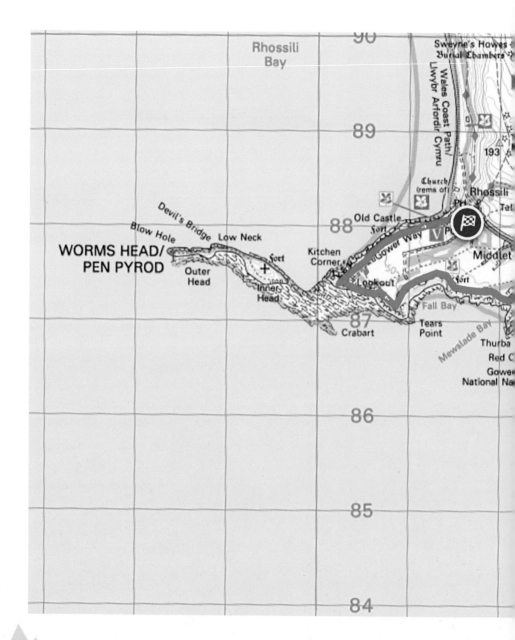

sea. It is around 1.6km (1 mile) long, and the causeway leading to it only emerges at low tide. From Worm's Head, follow the popular path into Rhossili and the end of your walk. This is a tourist area, so there are pubs and cafes from which to buy refreshments.

Take time to enjoy the magnificent golden arc of Rhossili beach before heading home.

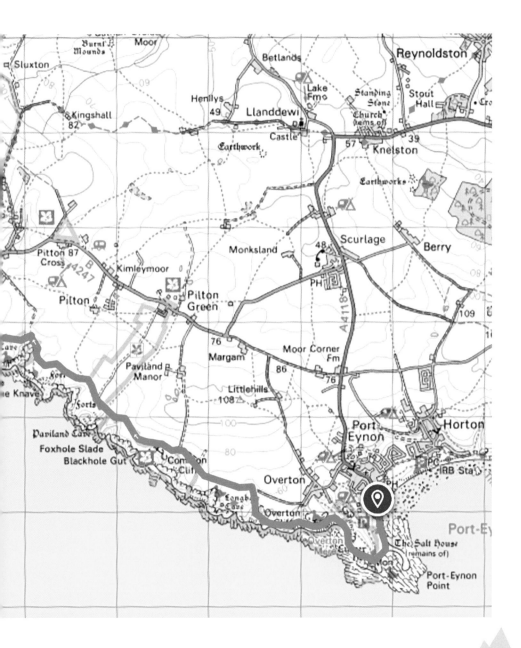

WALK 7:

RAVENSCAR TO ROBIN HOOD'S BAY CIRCULAR WALK

Enjoy the national park in a nutshell on this 17.7km (11-mile) walk through some of the North York Moors' most characteristic landscapes, starting and finishing at Ravenscar National Trust Coastal Centre. From the craggy heights of Ravenscar, the route runs across Howdale Moor before dropping down to the old Scarborough-to-Whitby railway line and along to the famous smugglers' haunt

of Robin Hood's Bay. Both here and at nearby Boggle Hole you can indulge in a spot of rock-pooling and fossil hunting, before returning along an exhilarating cliff-top stretch of the Cleveland Way National Trail, via the old alum works industrial site.

Walk down the concrete track in front of Ravenscar National Trust Coastal Centre. Go straight on at signs marked

Description: More than a beginner's hike, there are steep steps and elevations

Distance: 17.7km (11 miles)/6.5 hours

Terrain: May be boggy underfoot in places

Toilets and refreshments: The Raven Hall Country House Hotel at Ravenscar has a bar and restaurant, and spectacular views from the gardens on the cliff top. There's also the Ravenscar Tearooms in the village. Robin Hood's Bay has several cafes, pubs and restaurants. Don't miss the cake at the cafe at Boggle Hole YHA – handily positioned for the Cleveland Way

Getting there by public transport: East Yorkshire Buses run from Scarborough to Ravenscar

Wooden steps lead down to the shore at Ravenscar, North Yorkshire. © Adobe Stock/Craig

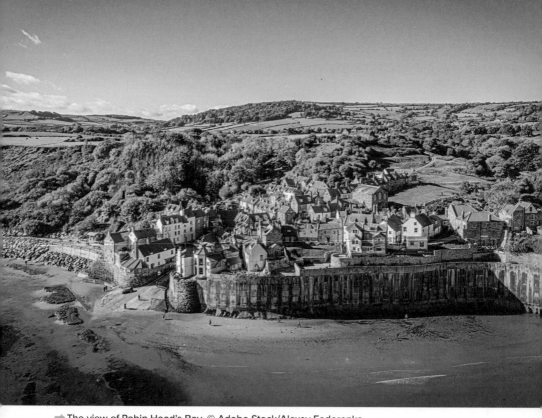

➡ The view of Robin Hood's Bay. © Adobe Stock/Alexey Fedorenko

'Trail' and 'Cleveland Way', then keep right at the 'Cleveland Way, Alum Works' sign.

At a 'Cleveland Way' signpost on your left, turn sharp left up a narrow path (signposted 'Public Footpath'). Shortly after crossing an old stone bridge, turn sharp right through a waymarked gate and follow the track up past Cragg Hall Farm. Turn right at the lane.

After the tarmac ends, continue along the track and cross the stile on your left. Bear right up the field towards the mast. Go through the gate at the top corner of the field and turn left. Cross the road and follow the bridleway over the moor.

At the crossroads of tracks, bear right along the bridleway (there's a waymarker post). Cross the road, follow the bridleway (Spring Hill), go through

the farmyard and then the gate. Bear left across the field. Turn right along the concrete track.

Turn right off the bridleway and immediately right again, through a gate, following the path uphill through Oxbank Wood – follow the waymarks as the path turns left, right and left again. Turn right, cross the stiles and keep straight on.

Bear right, over a stile (signposted 'Howdale') and cross another stile to reach a minor road at a bend. Turn left, downhill, and follow the road as it hairpins around the house. Below the house, turn right, through two high wooden kissing gates. Keep the fence on your left and follow the path into the wood.

Cross the bridge and stile and go straight over the field.

Cross the stone stile, turn left, then turn right into woods and over a wooden bridge. Continue ahead, across a sloping shale tip, then past a house and along the track. At the Trekking Centre, turn left through the first gate (through stone gateposts), walk down through the yard and turn left on to the old railway line.

At the farm, turn right over the stile (signposted 'Footpath to Beach'). In Robin Hood's Bay, turn right up Flagstaff Steps and then left along the cliffs to Boggle Hole and Stoupe Beck Sands. (If the tide's out you can walk along the shore instead.)

Cross the footbridge over Stoupe Beck and turn right uphill, following the Cleveland Way – first along a country lane and then left along a footpath ('Ravenscar 2 miles').

Turn left at the 'Cleveland Way, Alum Works' signpost. Continue, then turn left at the 'Cleveland Way' sign and return to Ravenscar.

More details and other free walks in the area are available from the North Yorkshire Moors National Park website (www.northyorkmoors.org.uk).

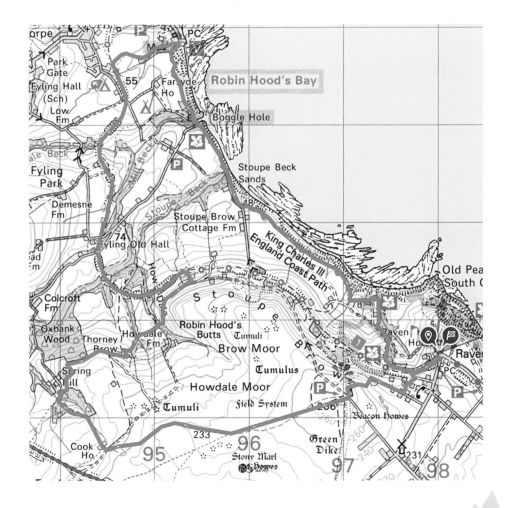

INTERVIEW: JO MOSELEY

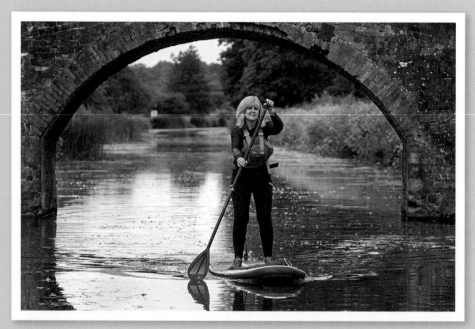

© Canal and River Trust

Jo: I'm Jo Moseley. I'm 58 and live in North Yorkshire and I am a mid-life adventurer. I write books, make many films, have a podcast called *The Joy of SUP – the Paddleboarding Sunshine Podcast* and do some creative consultancy. I also work for a church as a parish administrator.

Rhiane: What do you do in the outdoors and how did you get started?

Jo: I paddleboard, I swim, I hike and I'm just getting back into camping. But what I think I do is I just find joy and peace in the outdoors. I found it after a really difficult time in my life when I was going through the perimenopause and I just sort of cracked open. Life became really difficult – I'd been through a divorce, my mum and dad were going through chemotherapy, and life just felt incredibly overwhelming.

And after an incident in Tesco, when I burst into tears in the middle of the supermarket, I took up indoor rowing as a friend suggested it might help me sleep. I also rediscovered the outdoors in terms of returning to swimming and hiking and then started paddleboarding. I just went back into the outdoors, which I'd loved as a young woman. I had sort of lost myself, really. So, I find joy and peace and community outdoors, and I also

find purpose because I litter pick every day and I'm an ambassador for the 2 Minute Foundation, a beach cleaning foundation.

Rhiane: You paddleboarded the length of the Leeds–Liverpool Canal and you made a film about it?

Jo: Yes, in 2019, I paddleboarded 261km (162 miles) from Liverpool to Leeds, and then from Leeds to Goole, so along the Leeds–Liverpool Canal and the Aire & Calder Navigation. Along the way, I was picking up litter and fundraising for the 2 Minute Foundation and The Wave Project, which is a surf therapy charity. The film, directed and produced by Frit Tam of Frit Films, is called *Brave enough: A journey home to joy*.

Then I wrote a book about beautiful places to paddleboard in England, Scotland and Wales, which went on to become a bestseller. In the summer of 2021, I went around the country just after lockdown and met lots of really lovely paddleboarders and experienced some amazing journeys. Now I'm now writing a book about paddleboarding in the Lake District.

" YOU'RE BRAVER THAN YOU BELIEVE. "

Rhiane: You said earlier that you'd broken down in Tesco. What made you feel like you had lost yourself?

Jo: I think nowadays women are encouraged to retain their identity as a woman in their own right, as well as being a mum and a partner, but my generation was encouraged to give up everything and almost lose ourselves in motherhood. And so I did, and then I was divorced. Suddenly, I was a single mum and I just lost my confidence. In my 20s, I'd kayaked in Alaska when I'd been at college in America, and I dived when I was at university in Scotland, but I had completely lost that love of the outdoors since then.

But, after losing my mum in 2013, I found that being in nature helped my grief massively. It was a place where I could find peace and a calm connection. Every time I stand on my paddleboard, I feel like a warrior – not a worrier! I feel a strength and confidence that I had just completely lost – and my natural default position is to worry. I always worry about everything!

Being in the outdoors allows me to strip back all the things that happen to you in life, things that make you think you're not good enough. I'm always going to be a mother. That's always going to be my most important and treasured role, along with daughter, sister and friend. (The wife thing didn't really work out for me!) But now I also have this other identity that the outdoors has given me, which is, you know, a paddleboarder, a swimmer, a hiker, a camper – all these different things. Now I'm a writer, a podcaster, a filmmaker, and before I didn't have that. Nature has nurtured me over the last few years.

Rhiane: That's beautiful. You've found your feet in loads of different ways in the outdoors, haven't you?

Jo: Yes, you know life changes and with divorce, you have to recalibrate and find your feet again. On a paddleboard, I find that strength. You find out who you are and let the criticisms that you faced in life sort of float away. I really have found my feet!

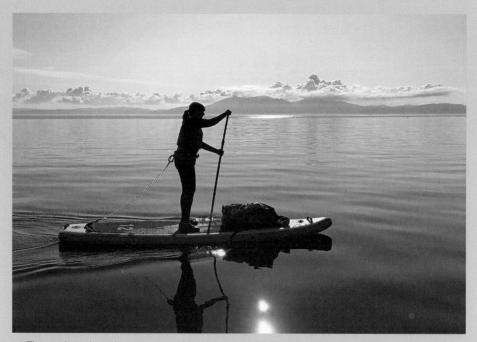

➡ The outdoors has given me a new identity as a paddleboarder. © Linn van der Zanden

Rhiane: As a mature woman, do you consider yourself to be a menopause advocate as well?

> **"**
>
> ## I JUST REALISED THAT LIFE IS VERY SHORT AND PRECIOUS. IF YOU'VE GOT THE SPARK OF A DREAM, YOU SHOULD GO FOR IT.
>
> **"**

Jo: The menopause broke me as I simply didn't know what was happening or that it was very much part of a stage in a woman's life, but it also broke me open and allowed other things to blossom. Nowadays, there's so much information that will make it easier for younger generations not to have to go through that confusion and pain, because they're much more knowledgeable. I want to advocate for the positives of the menopause in terms of looking after yourself, refocusing, recalibrating, finding out who you are again. The menopause kind of stopped me in my tracks and made me re-evaluate who I was.

Now I think about healthy ageing and what it means to be an older woman, ageing well, and how the outdoors can really benefit that. And one thing I've really noticed recently, particularly in my research in the Lakes, is that there are so many women in their 60s, 70s and 80s in the outdoors. They are there just quietly walking the fells, swimming the lakes, paddleboarding, and camping. They're so inspiring.

And I sort of see that the outdoors is an amazing place for women to age, to live and age bravely and I just love it. I see older women in the lakes just doing their thing, it's so very uplifting.

Rhiane: What kind of challenges do you feel that you face as an older woman in the outdoors?

Jo: I think many of the challenges were within myself, the sense that maybe I was being selfish taking time away for myself when I had my boys and dad to look after. I had grown up believing that I shouldn't put myself first. I think younger women are much better at realising they should.

I mean, I'm a white middle-class woman who grew up in the countryside so I have many, many privileges. I'm very aware of that. But when I first put the idea out there to paddleboard coast to coast, I would get comments that I couldn't do it – that it would be boring, too much for a woman of my age and logistically complex. So, I put the idea away for three years. In that intervening period, my son went off to university and I lost a number of girlfriends – only one of them had reached 50. And I just realised that life is very short and precious. If you've got the spark of a dream, you should go for it.

But even when I was on the canal, there was that small element of people deliberately undermining me. After asking me where I'd been, one chap said, 'In your dreams' – he just didn't believe I'd paddled 113km (70 miles). Another said, 'When you fall in, you'll get Weil's disease!' People underestimate older women; society undermines older women, and we're very easily dismissed – even with all the privileges I have.

Rhiane: Definitely. Do you think it's how society is conditioned to view women?

Jo: I don't think it was a surprise that those comments came from middle-aged men! And yet there were many who were really lovely. But remember, four years ago, not many people had seen many paddleboarders. Now they wouldn't bat an eyelid. But women would ask me questions about paddleboarding and how they might learn, which was wonderful.

I never consider that I inspire anyone – it's not something that I feel comfortable saying about myself. Somebody said to me that my superpower is my ordinariness. I'm relatable, just utterly normal and ordinary. I do like to think I might be an encourager, a cheerleader. And people can think, *Well if she can do that, maybe there's something I can do*. It might sow a tiny little seed of hope, then they go and do a Parkrun, or they go for a swim or a hike. It's never about saying, 'Look at what I can do.' It's about saying, 'What might you do that brings you joy and lifts your soul?'

And that's the message I try to convey, because the outdoors has given me so much. I don't need to look at Instagram for inspiration, I just go to the Lakes and I see all these women hiking and swimming and I'm just like, *wow*! Women who have known each other for ages, going out and living their best lives in their 60s, 70s and 80s. It's just amazing. I feel like I'm just getting started when I am around them.

Rhiane: Well really you are, there is no limit in the outdoors for anything.

Jo: I recently paddled with Debbie North, who is a wheelchair user and an inspirational champion for access to the outdoors for all. We had an amazing and very special weekend together paddleboarding in the Lakes. I truly believe there is a place for all of us in the outdoors where we can be free of judgement.

Rhiane: If you could give a bit of advice to somebody about finding their feet in the outdoors, what would you say?

Jo: I would say, 'Find what brings you joy.' Just follow your curiosity, and if it goes down one route and you're like, 'Well, this isn't really my thing,' just do something else. There's no time limit. Nobody's judging you. It's completely on your terms. It's your journey, you don't need to rush into things or to do big challenges.

If you could possibly pick up some litter, that would be good too! The environment has given me so much, I want to say thank you. It's as simple as that.

And find a community. I'm not a massively 'groupy' person. I like doing things on my own or with two or three other people, but you can find a community that you can dip in and out of, or you might have a virtual community online. I always love your stories, Rhiane! I am always wondering, *Where is she now? What's she doing?* I feed off that.

You know, life is so short. I'm 58 and I'm very aware of people my age who are dying now, or dying in their 60s or 70s. I'm just getting started but I'm also very aware that life ends at some point, and I want to make the most of it, not put my dreams off.

Rhiane: And do you feel fulfilled now, in everything that you're doing?

Jo: Yes, I do. Sometimes I get stressed, but I do feel fulfilled. I feel like the outdoors is a place that I can just keep learning and growing in. It's opened up so many opportunities for me. And, like Winnie the Pooh said, 'You're braver than you believe.'

66
I TRULY BELIEVE THERE IS A PLACE FOR ALL OF US IN THE OUTDOORS WHERE WE CAN BE FREE OF JUDGEMENT.
99

INTERVIEW: STEPH DWYER _____

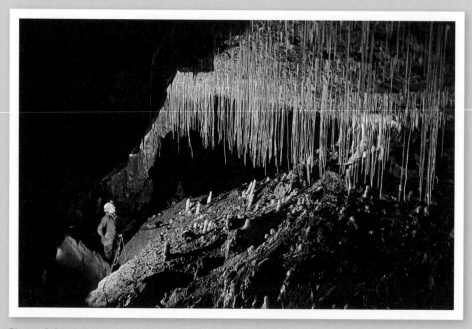

Photos © Steph Dwyer

Steph: My name is Steph Dwyer. I am 39 years old and I'm the managing director of an outdoor education centre, Yorkshire Dales Guides. I am also now a trainee clinical psychologist. I live in Settle in the Yorkshire Dales, but I'm originally from Ireland.

Rhiane: Can you tell me a little bit about your role at Yorkshire Dales Guides?

Steph: We basically do all sorts of outdoor adventure activities and training courses. We specialise in using the outdoors and nature as a therapeutic tool to help folk manage trauma and soothe the effects of chronic stress. I love working with underprivileged groups. Trauma is carried in the body. It is about giving participants the tools they need to overcome their hard-wired, physical responses to stress.

Rhiane: And how did you get into outdoor adventuring?

Steph: I think I probably got a real love for the outdoors from my dad. I come from a working-class family, so doing outdoor activities for fun

was not my introduction. My parents didn't have time for leisure, they were working all the time. But it was different when we went on summer holidays. Both sides of my family are farmers and so we would go down to County Clare, where my mum is from, which is an absolutely stunning region where I tried surfing and watersports.

Then we would go to my dad's family in County Sligo on the west coast and I would be constantly outdoors there, working on the farm and having fun. And then we would get four days away to this incredible island off the west coast, called Achill Island. It's my favourite place in the entire universe. There are beaches and mountains and I would be in the water the whole time.

Then I went to Dublin City University, which had loads and loads of outdoor clubs. But they didn't have a surf club. And I remember seeing this guy hanging from a rope in the ceiling at the freshers' fair. And I just thought, *That looks so cool*, and I went up and joined, not really knowing what club he was from. I was mortified to find I'd joined the caving society!

But I went along. It was terrifying, but mysterious. I almost wasn't going to go again, but one of the guys from the club said, 'Actually, you're not half bad at this, you know.' And I reluctantly went on the second trip, but mostly because he was really good-looking.

Rhiane: How did you know caving was for you?

66
I HAVE SO MUCH MORE STRENGTH THAN I EVER IMAGINED.
99

Steph: I realised that, once the fear had subsided, I could experience an entirely different world. The first time I was just afraid and my brain was saying, *Let's just survive this*. But once I got over that, I had this entirely different experience of the same places, and that was really mind-blowing. It was such a mindblowing experience for me, and I've taken it through my work to this very day. I think that informs a lot of my practice as a psychologist and as someone who uses psychology as a tool to help kids think differently about themselves and their world and build their self-esteem.

Rhiane: So how many years have you been caving for now?

Steph: I'm 39 now, and I've been caving since I was 18 years old. But when I grew up in working-class Ireland, there was no such thing as people having loads of hobbies in their spare time, especially hobbies that cost money. That would be considered frivolous.

Rhiane: It's like when our parents came to Britain. They came here to work, and having hobbies is very much a privilege, especially if you have caring responsibilities or lack free time and financial resources.

Steph: Yeah, it was just not a privilege people had. When I was a kid, the attitude to caving was very much like, 'We should understand that from a geological perspective,' not because it was fun!

Rhiane: What are your main achievements in caving?

Steph: I was the first Irish woman to bottom a 1,000-metre (3,281-feet)-deep cave. Looking at it through a feminist lens, once I had broken that psychological barrier, loads of other women did it after me, which was really cool. And then I was the first woman incident commander and underground controller for the world's oldest and busiest team in the Cave Rescue Organisation.

I am also a founder of the Ario Caves Project, which has won multiple awards, and was originally run by Oxford University Cave Club. Now, I've done loads of 1,000-metre (3,281-feet)-deep caves and I've also been the first person to find some new caves, which is really cool.

Some of the achievements that mean the most to me are what it's taken for me, as a woman, to carve my own sense of identity as a female caver and a female leader. And what it's taken mentally, psychologically and physically to make it to the bottom of some really, really deep holes in the ground. And finally, what it's required of me as a member of a team, being part of a community of people who put a common goal first.

The Ario Caves Project is based in the Picos de Europa in north-west Spain. We were the subject of Paul Diffley's film, *The Ario Dream*, about our aim to document one of the world's deepest cave systems. The Picos are mountains where there is no water on the surface. All the water is underground in a vast network of caves. We go out there every year, though Oxford University Cave Club have been going out here there since the 1950s.

We're so lucky to be going out exploring this virgin limestone and finding new caves that have never been seen by another human being.

Rhiane: You're literally going where no one's been before?

Steph: Yes! All cavers are part of an understated group of people who just quietly go about doing all this amazing stuff under the radar. You come out of an entrance of a cave and you haven't seen daylight for five days and you've barely slept, and you've just done one of the most extraordinary physical and mental feats of your life. But there are no medals, there's no trophy. It's just this profoundly deep experience that's happened between you and this environment and I just love that.

Rhiane: I think you do only hear about the people who have, say, done Everest because the more privileged activities get more press attention.

Steph: And the thing I like about that is it doesn't matter because cavers don't give a f***. It's not about the ego for them. My personal experience is that it's very much a deeply spiritual experience. I have had some of the

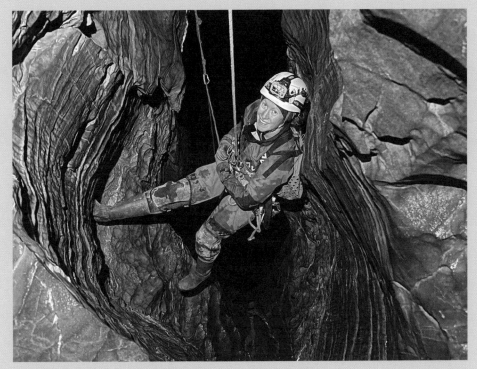

➡ Caving means being part of a team who put a common goal first.

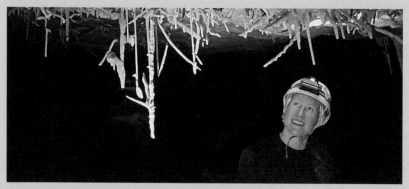
➡ Caving can be breathtakingly beautiful.

most transcendental experiences. I'm not religious at all, but I definitely feel there is something bigger to all of this. You just feel so humble.

Mine might be the very first footprint that has been left in that sand or left in that mud, or yours are the first eyes that have seen something that is hundreds of thousands of years old. It is a breathtakingly beautiful, deeply personal thing.

Rhiane: That must be so inspiring. Have there been any single, specific events that have been challenging, life-altering or have really shifted your perspective?

Steph: Yes, when I was on an Ario expedition in 2013, I was 550 metres (1,805 feet) underground, and I had been underground for five days doing a big exploration trip. It was near the end and I was really, really tired when I was coming back out and had a really bad fall. I could have died. In the end, I broke my scaphoid [a bone in the wrist], dislocated my thumb and chipped some of the bone off it, broke some bones in my foot and tore my meniscus [cartilage] in my knee. I was incredibly lucky to be alive. But there's no helicopter to come and save you, so I had to self-rescue out of the cave because if I'd stayed and laid there and waited for rescue, I would have succumbed to hypothermia.

So, with the help of a couple of friends, I had to get up a 140-metre (460-feet)-high waterfall. I had to go directly up the rope to get to the top of this with broken bones. You would imagine that that would be something that would be harrowing and impossible. But the thing that was really extraordinary to me was that I got myself out, and it was actually this deeply empowering experience.

Rhiane: Wow. Wow, that is insane.

Steph: But it showed me the extraordinary strength and tenacity that I had, and that things are probably never as bad as in your imagination. It showed me how incredibly lovely friends can be and how people can really step up to a situation. It really changed me a lot because it actually gave me a huge amount of confidence. You would expect someone to be traumatised and never want to go back into a cave again. And it definitely showed me how vulnerable I was. It took us 14 hours to get out. But I had so much strength, so much more than I imagined.

Rhiane: What do you think about in terms of diversity and inclusion and creating equity in the outdoor space. What have you noticed? What have you seen change and what would you like to see?

Steph: Yeah. So this is something that's really important to me. I think there is very little diversity within caving. And I think that's a function of privilege. A lot of these expeditions are really, really costly and time-consuming. Also, a lot of caving clubs were university clubs historically. There are two things you need: money and a job where you can get a lot of time off, and we know that those privileges are disproportionately held by white folks.

Of course, there's not a huge amount of diversity there in terms of race, but there is diversity in loads of other ways. There's a lot of neurodiversity in caving, and queer and gender-fluid folk are just completely and utterly accepted for who they are. It's just not diverse along the axis of colour.

I really miss this, and it's because of the experiences that I've had with you BGH ladies. You have an incredibly tough and really great 'can-do' attitude that I just don't see as much in white communities. I just think that the caving community would hugely benefit from diversity.

I'm not 100 per cent sure, but I don't think there would be that much actual racism within the community. So, I think what we need to do is address the systemic reasons why people of colour are not accessing the outdoors and create a safe, welcoming space for folk to participate.

66

I THINK WHAT WE NEED TO DO IS ADDRESS THE SYSTEMIC REASONS WHY PEOPLE OF COLOUR ARE NOT ACCESSING THE OUTDOORS AND CREATE A SAFE, WELCOMING SPACE FOR FOLK TO PARTICIPATE.

99

Rhiane: I really like what you said about different types of diversity, because I think at the moment there seems to be a focus on skin colour, which can be a bit 'box-ticky'. I also think that within an all-white group you might hear casual racism, and if you don't at all, that's really positive. But then caving doesn't seem as hierarchical as other sports.

Steph: The value system against which you're measured just doesn't go along any of those quotients. It's very much about who you are as a person, 'Are you someone who's team-oriented? Are you going to pull your weight?' Because there was always this expectation that I could carry the same as everyone else, so I just picked up the kit and carried it.

It has no hierarchy. And you know, though I've experienced loads of sexism in my life, I've not experienced it in caving. It's just a case of, we're all the same when we're caked head to toe in mud! It's not an issue. We've recently had a friend of ours who's come out as trans and we've just carried on as normal.

When I got older, I thought, *Hold on a minute*. What society is telling me about my capability and what is actually happening here are two totally different things. I now think, *Of course I can do this!* because on every other trip, I do the same as the boys, so why when I go down a 1,000-metre (3,281-feet)-deep cave would it be any different? I think that's my favourite thing about the caving community: people can absolutely, truly, be themselves.

Rhiane: What's the one thing you would say to someone who is maybe struggling to get into adventure? How do they find their feet?

Steph: The one thing I would say to folk is, if you don't see somebody like yourself in the outdoors, don't be afraid to go out and pave your own path. Don't wait until you feel ready. You will only find your limits if you're prepared to push them, and you have to be prepared to fail, so don't be afraid of failure. This requires you to cultivate and realise a deep sense of your own worthiness.

If you get to know and love yourself, you will find that you are probably way more capable than you think you are. If you were to talk to the little child I was, and see what low self-esteem I had, you would never in a million years think that very shy, insecure little girl is the person I am now.

Explore, take chances, take risks, take failure as a measure of bravery and courage, and go out and just flipping enjoy yourself!

WALK 8:

SENNEN COVE AND LAND'S END

The coastal scenery around Cornwall's western tip is stunning: rocky and wild, with seas that churn a turbulent blue and white in windy weather (and are still considered dangerous for boats). Sea birds are numerous, and though Land's End is a famous landmark and attracts many visitors, you don't have to walk far along the South West Coast Path to experience vast and beautiful expanses of beach, and open, endless skies.

Of course, you could drive to Land's End, the westernmost point in the country, and pay for parking in what looks like a small theme park of cafes, shops and attractions – and there's nothing wrong with that, if that's your bag. But if you take this walk from Whitesands Bay at Sennen Cove, you'll approach Land's End from the magnificent coastal path. This walk offers spectacular views, wildlife and historical interest. In spring, the cliffs are alive with nesting fulmars, kittiwakes and guillemots and the cliff tops are covered in wild flowers. Secluded Nanjizal Beach is dog-friendly and very beautiful.

There are two pay-and-display car parks at Sennen Cove, one at each end of the village. Both are likely to be busy in the summer. Start at the beach car park at the southern end of Whitesands

Description: Moderate, some steep climbs and rough surfaces

Distance: 5.3km (3.3 miles)/1.5 hours

Terrain: Varied – grassy, surfaced roads and unfenced clifftops

Toilets and refreshments: Several pubs and cafes in Sennen Cove. Land's End has lots of facilities

Getting there by public transport: Regular bus services from Penzance, St Ives and St Just to Sennen Cove and Land's End

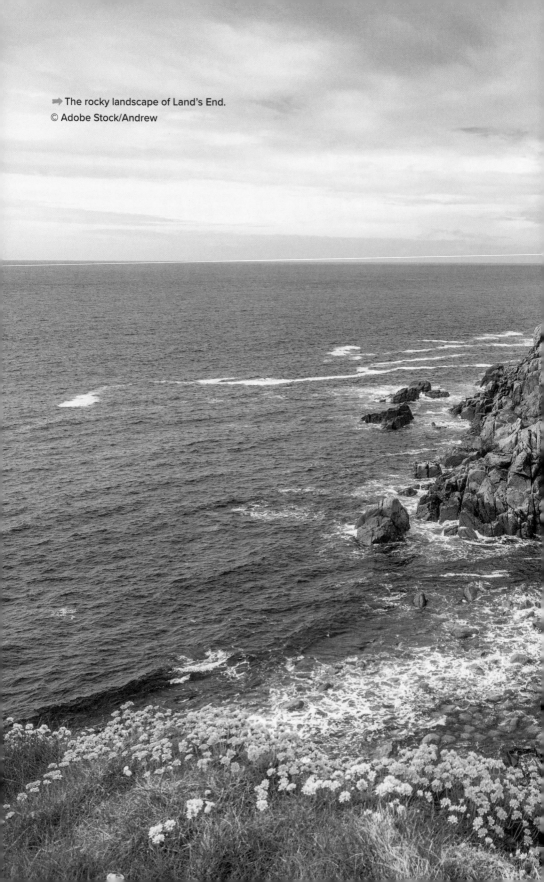

The rocky landscape of Land's End.
© Adobe Stock/Andrew

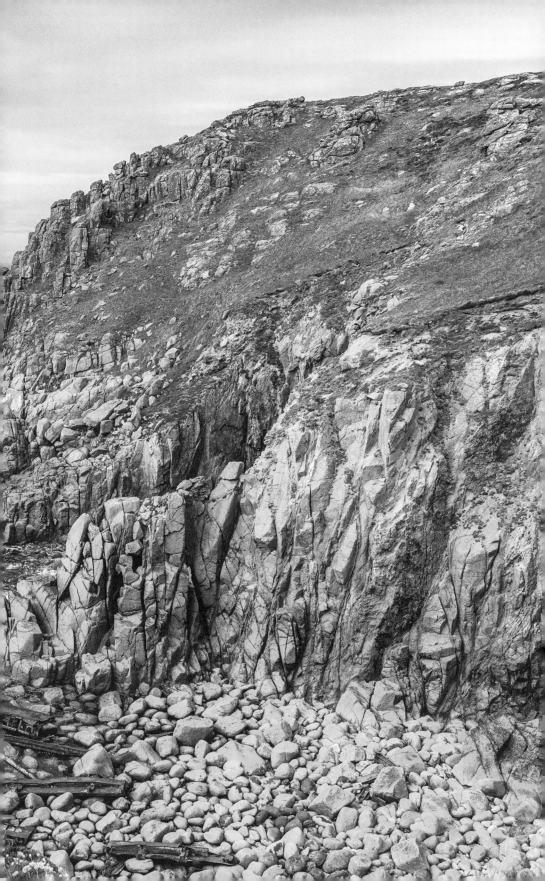

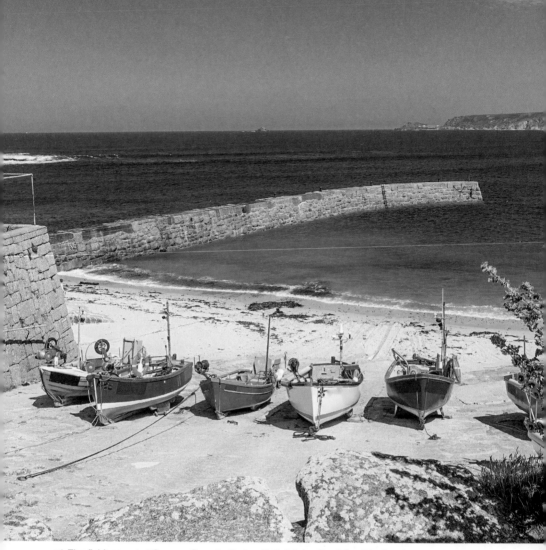

➡ The fishing port at Sennen Cove in Cornwall. © Adobe Stock/Ian Woolcock

Bay. Sennen Cove still has a small fishing fleet and a few pleasure boats, but the sea is dangerous (the first lifeboat was stationed here in 1853). Head up the road and turn first right to walk along the top of the village and take in the lovely views.

The lane will turn left, but you will keep walking straight on, travelling inland, following the footpath across fields and making for a house you can see on the horizon. This is Treeve Moor House. Keep walking straight ahead, until you meet the A30 road. Cross it (taking care) and carry on walking along the B3315 road towards Trevescan.

Keep going until you see the Little Barn Cafe, then turn right. You will pass through a garden and climb a stile. Keep walking along the left side of the fields, to cross the farmyard at Trevilley, over a stile and on to a track, where you should turn right.

The track will end and you should follow footpath signs through three fields

FINDING YOUR FEET

until you reach a gate at the edge of a valley. Turn right again here and this narrow path will descend steeply to the coastal path that runs above Nanjizal, or Mill Bay as it's also known. To access the beach, turn left on the path, then bear right. As this beach is only accessible by foot, it is typically deserted, with no cafe or car park to bring the crowds. Planning a picnic here would be a fantastic idea on a sunny day!

Return to the coast path and follow the rocky route along the back of the bay before climbing up on the edge of Trevilley Cliff. Follow the cliff edge round to Pordenack Point. If you're lucky, you may spot seals here, but you'll definitely pass interesting rock formations, including a rock arch just off the coast.

As the path approaches Land's End, it becomes increasingly worn. Keep following the coast path signs nearest to the cliffs. Glebe Farm will be on your right until you follow the signposted steps down and uphill to eventually reach the Land's End official signpost.

From here, follow the coast path over Maen Cliff and you'll soon see the remains of the iron age fort of Maen Castle. The National Trust has restored the old coastguard lookout up here and there are fabulous views down to Whitesands Bay, where you started your journey.

Then drop down to Sennen Cove and explore the harbour and the shops there before walking along the beachfront back to the car park.

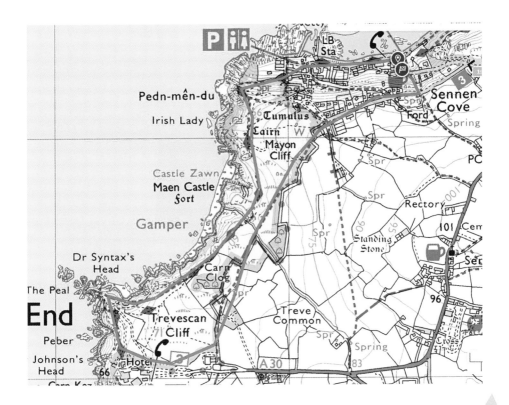

INTERVIEW: YVETTE CURTIS

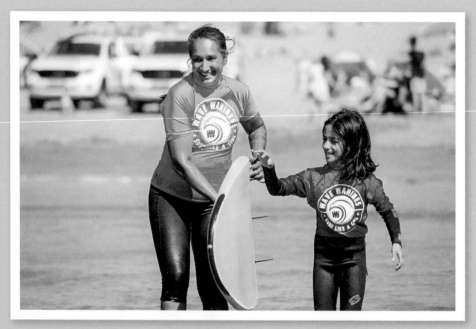

Photos © Yvette Curtis

Yvette: I'm Yvette Curtis and I live in North Devon, just outside of Croyde. I used to be a personal trainer. Then I started a surf club, Wave Wahines. Now I'm an equality, diversity and inclusion manager.

Rhiane: What is your background in the outdoors?

Yvette: As a kid, I always loved sports. And when it came to A-levels, part of them involved outdoor-related pursuits. So, I did kayaking, climbing and canoeing, all that stuff. As an adult, my eldest child wanted to go surfing, and I love being outdoors and being by the sea, and it took off from there.

Rhiane: So, tell me a bit about Wave Wahines.

Yvette: When we looked at the local community and the local provider for my child's lessons, it was really expensive, over £35 for a session. I was a self-employed personal trainer, so it was never going to happen! The local clubs were also quite exclusive, quite closed. They were for people who already had their own equipment and some surfing knowledge. So I thought we could try to create one, and I spoke to a couple of female

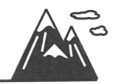

coaches who I knew at a local surf school and we decided to give it a go.

I thought I couldn't be the only parent of a child who doesn't come from a surfing background but wants to learn the sport, and to learn about the ocean. We're a coastal community, so it's important to have that knowledge as well, just as a life skill. So we created it on a whim. And luckily the surf school was supportive and let us use their kit for a year to make it cost-effective. I just had to pay for the coaches. We tried to keep it as cheap as possible. When we started seven years ago it was £10 a session, and we haven't changed it — it's still £10.

Rhiane: What groups of people do you work with?

> # 66
> # I KEPT HEARING THAT SURFING IS REALLY ACCESSIBLE AND I THOUGHT, *NO IT'S NOT!*
> # 99

Yvette: It's women and girls from our local community. Our first event was free, and over 20 women and girls turned up, so we knew there was an appetite for it. We deliver surf sessions, but we also have a winter programme, so we keep our girls together doing things like roller skating, skateboarding, trampolining and jewellery making. We'll have movie nights and go to the local countryside and do creative art sessions.

But in surf culture, I was quick to realise there weren't many faces like mine looking back at me. There may be three or four women out of 20 people in a room, but I was always the only person of colour. And I just thought, why is that?

Then, when George Floyd was murdered, it was a point of reflection for all industries and surfing was no different. Suddenly, there were calls from every part of the press and the media to ask: 'Why is surfing so un-diverse?' I didn't want to represent all people of colour, all ethnicities, all cultures — I was really uncomfortable with it — but equally, someone needed to speak. So many times I heard people say that surfing is such an accessible sport and I thought, *Oh, it's really not!* I don't think that comment was ever made out of malice, it's just a lack of knowledge. People don't see the barriers if they don't exist for *them*. But that doesn't mean they don't exist for other people.

> ## 66
> ## PEOPLE DON'T SEE THE BARRIERS IF THEY DON'T EXIST FOR *THEM*. BUT THAT DOESN'T MEAN THEY DON'T EXIST FOR OTHER PEOPLE.
> ## 99

I said, there *are* barriers, and it can be a really difficult sport to get into. So three years ago we ran a diversity and surf group not knowing how the community would respond, and who might want to participate. And we certainly weren't expecting the community we got, which was young female Syrian refugees. We surfed with six families that had been displaced and resettled here. That group's been running for three years now. It's shown such growth and the girls are fantastic.

Equally, it's been a challenge to our working practices because, while we were ready to look at different communities and cultures, we suddenly had the language barrier to deal with. We also encountered massive trauma because of what those young people had witnessed during the war. It was challenging for us, but it's been the most rewarding work. It's been incredible.

We also work with women who are living in refuge from domestic violence. So, we are reaching really, really different communities that normally would not be exposed to surfing for one reason or another, whether it's geographically, financially or just a lack of feeling like they belong. The surf industry is definitely still quite a white space, but it is changing. There's still a lot of work to do.

Rhiane: That's fantastic. BGH has just been funded to reach hidden communities.

Yvette: That's amazing. I don't think we realised the impact we could have just by reaching out. We've worked with Reclaim The Sea in Plymouth as well, and they're doing really similar stuff. We've been to community evenings where we've had Syrian food, and we also ensure that our surf sessions don't run over Ramadan. That's the whole point of being inclusive: to make sure you're respecting everybody's religion and culture.

Rhiane: And you mentioned that you're doing equality, diversity and inclusion work now. What kind of organisations are you working with and what have been your successes and challenges?

Yvette: Surfers Against Sewage advertised a completely new position as an equality, diversity and inclusion manager with them to help shape and drive their entire organisational strategy. And I just thought, you know what, I'm going to apply for this one. I thought of it as my last shot as, despite having applied for similar things within this space and being invited to talk and write articles, I didn't get a job with a place at the decision-making table. But I got the role!

I've come up against some quite challenging moments regarding the governance structures within English surfing. It feels like there's a real defensiveness, with people not wanting to talk about diversity and not wanting to actually change things, or even just recognise and acknowledge the issues. So those have been major barriers, but I have

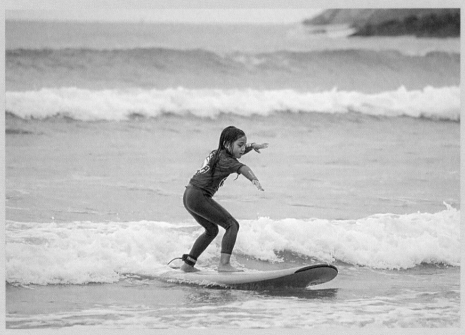

➡ Working towards making surfing inclusive.

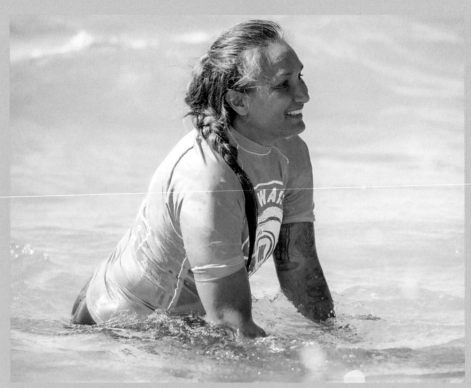
➡ Feeling connected and grounded in the water.

just kept knocking on that door and just saying there is an issue here
with conservation spaces and with surf spaces. Now, it's great to be in an
organisation that is open to change, isn't afraid to put themselves out there
and actually isn't afraid to make mistakes. They know there's work to do,
and they're going to do it as authentically as they can. At my interview I
just said, 'Do you mean this or is this just to secure more funding?' I've left
organisations and I've taken our club away from organisations because they
lacked integrity. But Surfers Against Sewage's answer was really honest.

I am really happy to be in a role where I'm helping to shape policy in
a space that crosses surfing, environmentalism and conservation, all of
which are massively underrepresented. I want to be one of those really
big championing voices ensuring marginalised communities have a space,
have a voice and are heard and seen at all levels of those organisations.

I have recently begun a body of work with GB Surfing, the overarching
organisation who will be aiming for the GB Olympic surfing team on how
we can shape their Diversity and Inclusion policies and strategies to
ensure we are getting the best surfers and not just the ones who currently
have access, as that may well be different.

I am also a core team member that brought the first UK World Surfing Reserve (of which there are only 12 worldwide) and we are ensuring 'Waves for all, Forever.'

Rhiane: What are your greatest successes?

Yvette: My greatest success is talking about this stuff in a really honest and I hope a really approachable manner. Getting the surf community to talk about it, to acknowledge it and to start covering it in their media. I hope my legacy is that I've played a small part in driving that change and driving that conversation.

Rhiane: Who do you admire in your sport?

Yvette: I'm a real fan of organisations like Sea Sisters and Arugam Bay Surf Club in Sri Lanka. They connect women and girls in those communities to the ocean. They deal with the major cultural barrier of girls' expected roles throughout their lives, which is so different to here. And I'd love to see more Wave Wahines clubs in other places, whether in the UK or overseas.

I really think it's so important that we're here. We're beginning to show a pathway of how to be in this industry, whether it's as an athlete or whether it's as a sports coach or whether it's as a commentator. At the moment that doesn't exist, and I'd really love to be a part of shaping that.

But systemic change takes so long, nothing's going to happen overnight. It just takes people who have got enough inner strength or enough support to just keep going.

Rhiane: How do you cope with activism? How do you stop yourself from getting burnt out?

Yvette: It's the sea. It's Mother Ocean. That's it for me. I always feel really connected and really grounded when I'm in the water. I have such a sense of calm, such a sense of connection and of who I am. So, I don't think my feelings for activism are going to change. I think I'll probably get more involved working at Surfers Against Sewage. My activism will probably grow. You know, I've got great support. I've got a great family and I want to protect the world for my three children. I've got my youngest, who is my colour, and I've got my eldest who is a member of the queer community. I'm fighting for marginalised communities and hoping to amplify their voices. I want to leave the world a better place.

WALK 9:

ST BEES CIRCULAR

Situated in a fairly secluded spot between Whitehaven and Egremont on the coast, St Bees has the only cliff tops in Cumbria, and is an extremely popular spot for walkers and bird lovers (there are several RSPB viewing spots along the cliff-top paths where it is possible to see guillemots, kittiwakes, fulmars and razorbills). On a clear day, the views may stretch as far as the Isle of Man. Dolphins and porpoises are found here and sandstone boulders are scattered along the beach, giving it a unique appearance.

This is a circular walk around St Bees Head and then on to Whitehaven that starts and finishes at Sea Mill car park in St Bees, returning on the England Coast Path (ECP) via Primrose Valley.

Start from the car park, which has a beautiful view of St Bees beach. At low tides, ancient peat beds with the remains of petrified trees can be seen. Look out for a life boat station and caravan park – you want to walk past these and over a bridge to South Head and the start of the cliff-top path (about 90 metres/100 yards away from the car park).

This cliff path is sandy and climbs quite steeply. The view in front of you will expand to show the beach and the village. Continue to follow the path around South Head until in front of you it begins to dip and the stony beach of Fleswick Bay comes into view. The path

Description: Easy/intermediate circular walk taking in both countryside and coastal scenery

Distance: 11.3km (7 miles)/2.5 hours

Terrain: Cliff-top path with some steep climbs; includes tracks and field paths that can be quite muddy after wet weather, as can the areas around some of the gates and stiles

Toilets and refreshments: Several pubs in the village

Getting there by public transport: By train, St Bees and Whitehaven are on the Cumbrian Coast Line. There are trains seven days a week

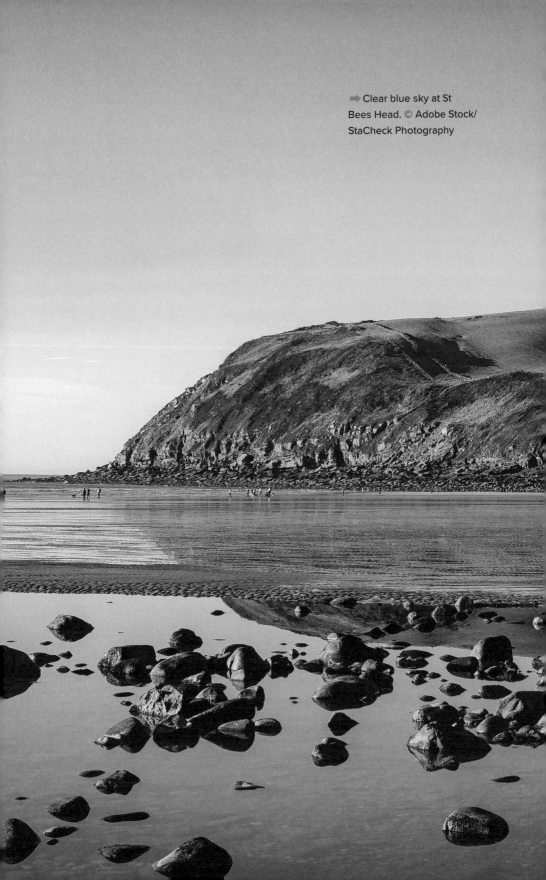

➡ Clear blue sky at St Bees Head. © Adobe Stock/ StaCheck Photography

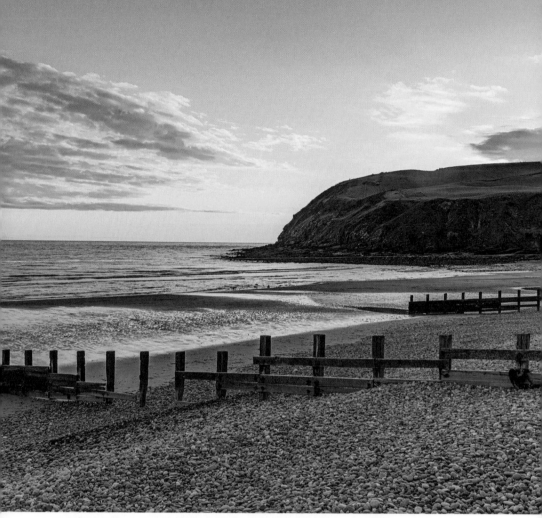

⮕ ABOVE: St Bees beach in Cumbria. © Adobe Stock/Bernd Brueggemann
⮕ OPPOSITE: St Bees Lighthouse on the coastal path. © Adobe Stock/makasana photo

will meet a junction from where you can take a slight detour on to the beach (be careful, this path can be slippery!).

Fleswick Bay is a fascinating destination in itself, as it was used by smugglers in the 19th century, who scratched their names into the wall of the cave you'll find in the cliffs. It is also famous for the semi-precious gemstones that wash up on the shore here. It's well worth stopping to comb the beach for an hour or so. Rejoining the cliff-top path, begin walking towards North Head, towards the pre-Victorian lighthouse

(built in 1822) that is still in use today. North Head is an RSPB reserve, with the nesting sites especially busy in spring. Its 300-metre (984-feet)-high cliffs are also popular with climbers.

Continuing north from the lighthouse, the path follows the boundary to the RSPB reserve until you reach a quarry, where you will turn away from the sea and follow the quarry access road back inland. You will reach a surfaced road that leads to a road junction.

Turn right at the road junction until you get to a crossroads. Carry on until

FINDING YOUR FEET

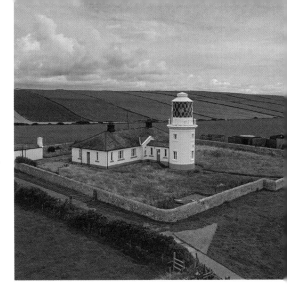

you see a signpost for Fleswick Bay and turn left here. This is Hannah Moor Lane. At the end of the lane, you will find four ladder stiles until the path goes diagonally across a field into its far corner (on the left).

Following the field boundary, the path takes you downhill to meet the waymarker above Fleswick Bay. From here, retrace your route back to St Bees beach and the car park.

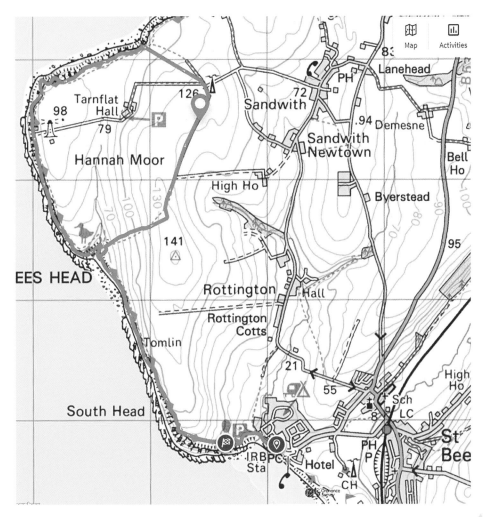

INTERVIEW: AMIRA PATEL

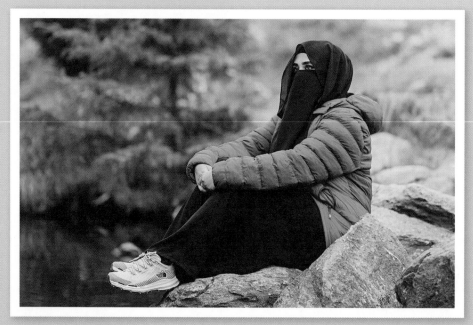

Photos © Amira Patel

Amira: I'm Amira Patel, 31, founder of The Wanderlust Women, an expedition leader and adventurer. I live in Cumbria.

Rhiane: What's your background in the outdoors?

Amira: Growing up I wasn't really into the same things as my friends, but my mum loved the outdoors, and she took my brother and I out horse-riding and hiking and things like that. I wasn't really very interested as a young teenager. On my first hike, I cried all the way, but I loved it when I got to the summit! So, when I was young, it was something that gave me time with my mum. Then I went on a backpacking trip when I was 21 and I found an adventurous side to me that I didn't know existed.

I rediscovered the outdoors after my divorce, when I decided to climb three mountains in England as a way to heal. After I went into the mountains, I reconnected with my faith in a really different way, and it showed me I was capable of achieving things. Sometimes, you need to be out of your comfort zone to realise who you are. You peel back all the layers of your personality and find out who you really are underneath. Now, this is my third year in the mountaineering world.

Rhiane: Why did you start The Wanderlust Women?

Amira: A career in the outdoors wasn't something I planned. It was a leap of faith, trusting in God and doing what I really loved. I started The Wanderlust Women as a side hustle, and only later did I start to get an income from it. It's grown through sheer determination and hard work. I had no knowledge of this field. If you really love something, you'll do everything to pursue it, you really just have to learn as you go. I achieved it through pure determination and working long hours.

66
I LOVE HELPING MUSLIM WOMEN TO CONNECT WITH THEIR FAITH, AND THEIR MENTAL AND PHYSICAL HEALTH.
99

Rhiane: What do you get from going on adventures?

Amira: Just getting outdoors has a massive impact on your mental, physical and spiritual health. For us, everything is centred around God and our faith. As long as I have that, the blessings and the doors that open are amazing. I love helping Muslim women to connect with their faith, mental health and physical health. We want to create a safe space, so they're around women who look like them. We create a community.

Rhiane: Are there ups and downs to running The Wanderlust Women?

Amira: Yes, people look up to me as a role model, but then they perceive I have everything, that my life is perfect. The downside is the trolls and the social media momentum. I manage it all through intention – I try to make my content meaningful. Most feedback is amazing, but there's that small number who want to give you crap. I just use them as motivation to continue.

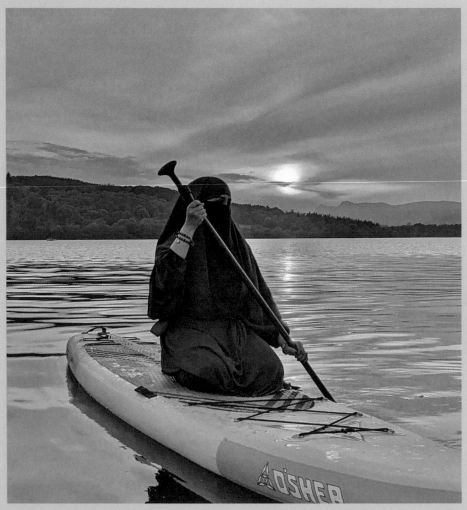

➡ Sometimes you need to get out of your comfort zone to realise who you are.

Rhiane: What do your family think of your career?

Amira: My family support everything I do. When I go home, my siblings have followed my journey. When you do something you love, and your family see that you're making it work, they're so proud.

Rhiane: What do you bring to your field?

> # SOMETIMES, YOU NEED TO BE OUT OF YOUR COMFORT ZONE TO REALISE WHO YOU ARE.

Amira: I definitely bring a new perspective, showing Muslim women are not just how the media portrays us. People see that this is us, we're not alien, there's nothing wrong with us. And this new perspective helps Muslim women feel valued and part of the space.

The outdoors gives me so much – I can't see a life without it. We all have our natural temperaments. I'm a person who belongs in nature, and I love helping people. So if I ever lose track of who I am, what I'm doing, I step out into the outdoors and I gain that clarity.

Just do it. You have to really believe: manifest it. Say out aloud, 'I am going to do this!' Write it down, look at it every day. And take the first step. If it works out, it works out, but if it doesn't, it doesn't, then you start again. It's not going to be easy, but once you see the ripple effect, it will be worth it. And for me, prayer is important.

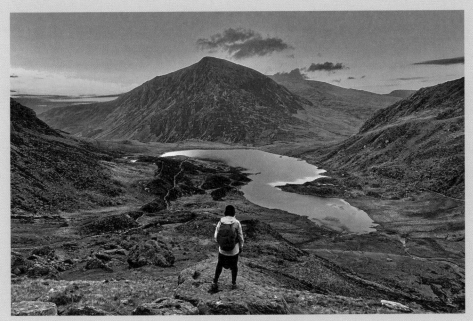

➡ The outdoors gives me so much – I can't see a life without it.

WALK 10:

THE PEAKS: MONYASH CIRCULAR

The Peaks are where I began my journey into the world of hiking – it was looking at the mysterious landscape through the train window that inspired me to hit the hills. This circular walk from the village of Monyash, following the Limestone Way in the Peak District, is an easy introduction to this gorgeous part of Britain. Passing through Cales Dale and Lathkill Dale, the area is characterised by the limestone walls of the White Peaks.

Monyash is a very pretty ancient Derbyshire village, about 11.3km (7 miles) from Buxton. This walk takes you out of the village and through part of Cales Dale, with its dramatic moss-covered trees, before following Lathkill Dale, through the open fields of Bagshaw Dale before returning to Monyash.

The walk starts on Rakes Road, opposite the village green. Walk away from the village, and you will pass a duck pond on your left.

From here, the road bears right, and you will follow it as it becomes a farm track. When the track also turns to the right, carry on along Milkings Lane (this has a signpost for the Limestone Way). On this path, you will pass through classic White Peak countryside, with its famous limestone walls.

Description: A beginner's hike, with steps and stiles, but no steep hills

Distance: 6.4km (4 miles)/2 hours

Terrain: Tracks, fields (some possibly muddy), some uneven ground and narrow gates

Toilets and refreshments: The Bulls Head or The Old Smithy cafe in Monyash

Getting there by public transport: Details of Peak District bus routes can be found at www.peakdistrict.gov.uk

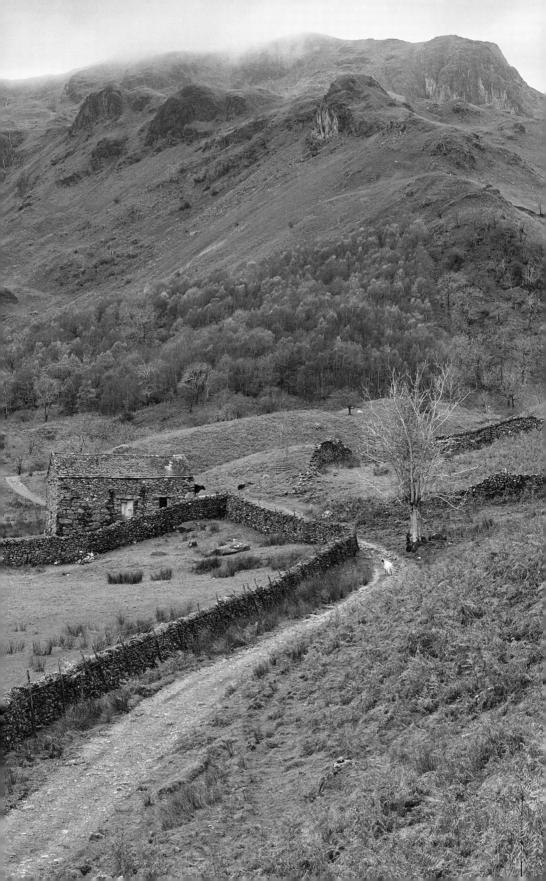

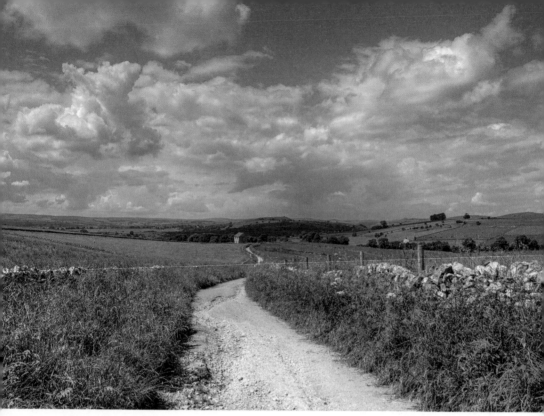

➡ ABOVE: A lane in White Peak, Hartington, Derbyshire. © Adobe Stock/Gail Johnson
➡ PAGE 209: Dovedale, near Buxton. © AdobeStock/S.R.Miller.jpeg

Continue on this path – there are paths off it but ignore these – until you reach a gate with a stile beside it. Carry on through the gate and through the next field, keeping to the left of the stone wall. You will see a sign for Fern Dale, and the path leads you through a gate in the stone wall (still signposted the Limestone Way).

Head diagonally across this field towards a small gate in the wall in front of you. Pass through this and walk through the next field, keeping to the right of the stone wall, still following the signs for the Limestone Way, and pass through another small gate followed by a stone stile after a short while. Continue on the path, to the left of the wall.

You'll get to a wide farm gate and here, ignore the signs for Lathkill Dale and instead go through the gate, turn left and follow the track back towards the buildings in front of you. You will encounter a path crossing yours but ignore this and carry straight on.

The track will fork in front of an old barn. Take the left-hand fork, signposted for Lathkill Dale, and pass a row of disused pigsties.

The track will soon fork again. This time, take the right-hand fork down towards a huddle of barns. There will be two barns in front of you and between them a gate and a path leading to some steps. Take these down into the field and follow the marked path through the field until you come to another gate. Go through the gate and follow the narrow track in front of you into Cales Dale. The path will pass to the right of a high rocky cliff. This is a really lovely spot!

FINDING YOUR FEET

You will meet a crossroads of paths and should turn left here to follow the signs for Lathkill Dale. This path twists and turns through some pretty woodland and passes the spot where a stream emerges from the ground, which eventually flows into the River Lathkill.

Carry on along this path until you reach a bridge over the River Lathkill. This is the entry to Lathkill Dale. Turn left here and follow the clearly marked path through the dale with the river on your left.

Look out for Lathkill Head Cave on your left. In wet weather, the River Lathkill flows into the dale from here.

The path continues through spectacular limestone cliffs, having now left the river. The path will become rocky and it can be slippery, and you will encounter a 'squeeze stile' before coming to a gate.

Go through the gate and straight through the open countryside and towards the road that you will eventually spot in front of you.

Cross the road and turn left, before almost straight away turning right just before some farm buildings. Keep to the left-hand side of a stone wall. Soon, the path will lead you to a stone stile and after this into another field.

From here, you carry on into Bagshaw Dale, walking through open countryside, keeping to the right of a stone wall. This easily followed path goes over another stone stile and a series of gates.

Eventually, you will encounter a squeeze stile at the side of a wider gate, and then join a quiet road. Turn left on the road and left again to walk back down into the village and the end of your circular walk.

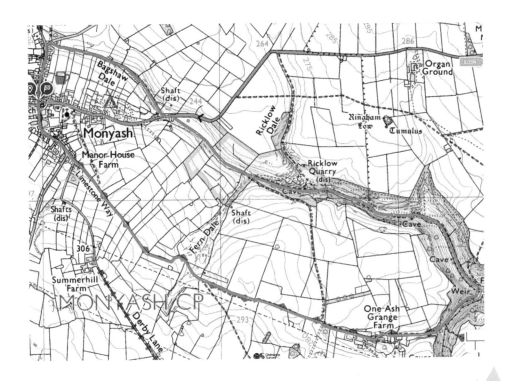

INTERVIEW: DEBBIE NORTH

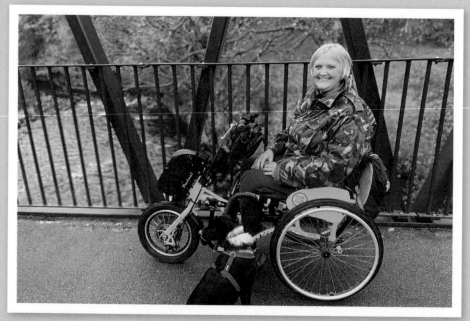

Photos © Debbie North

Debbie: I'm Debbie North. I'm 61, Yorkshire born and bred, and I live on the edge of the Yorkshire Dales National Park. I'm a consultant, writer and speaker specialising in access to the countryside.

Rhiane: And how did you get into adventuring?

Debbie: Since I was a little girl, I have always been outdoors. My dad said I should have been born in a field! I had an inspirational teacher at school called Mr Fletcher, who got me into orienteering and camping, and we used to go up to the school farm in the Peak District. So I really nurtured that love of being in the outdoors and that continued when I met Andy, my husband. We spent our holidays doing either long-distance walks or exploring the Yorkshire Dales and the Lake District, and we fell in love with walking.

Rhiane: How did you become an accessibility advocate?

Debbie: In 2009, I started getting backache and an MRI showed that I had degeneration of the spine. My consultant said, 'I don't even know how you're still standing with the state of your spine,' and I ended up being

a wheelchair user. But I didn't want to let my love of the outdoors fade, simply because I was in a wheelchair.

I put out a blog called *Access the Dales*. I remember writing the blog on 28 February 2011, and it basically said, 'Who am I?' I was no longer a head teacher — I had to give up due to ill health. I had been head of a primary school, and I loved working with children. I was no longer the mum that I used to be because my son had grown up and was off to university. I started exploring all-terrain wheelchairs when I didn't even know what one was.

> ## " I CAN'T BELIEVE THAT THERE ARE PEOPLE WHO CAN'T GET OUT BECAUSE THEY'VE GOT A DISABILITY. "

The response I got from that first blog was immense. The number of people who wrote in and said, 'I know exactly how you're feeling, and I know how it's so difficult to get outdoors.' So, Andy and I raised money for the first all-terrain wheelchair in the Yorkshire Dales National Park. It is still going strong up at Malham Tarn — we gifted it to the National Trust so people can have a wonderful walk around Malham.

Then we started having adventures. We linked up with a company called TerrainHopper who make wheelchairs that are the equivalent of my four seasons hiking boots, and my goodness, it was a life changer. I was back up on the mountains again, really pushing the barriers of mobility and disability in the hills, back on top of Skiddaw or Blencathra, where people would say, 'How have you got up here?'

Rhiane: What did you do next?

Debbie: In 2015, I did the coast to coast again, which is a special long-distance walk close to my heart. The first time I walked it, I fell in love with Andy. The second time I walked it, Andy proposed to me and the third time I did it, it was in a wheelchair and the start of my new career. It's how I became a consultant and an expert in how to get people outdoors into the countryside. And life was bloody good then, we were having so many adventures. It was just wonderful.

Then, two years ago, Andy passed away, which left me broken-hearted. So began a grieving process that I'm still going through. I'm on my own now. I'm living with a disability. He did all the driving; he lifted all my wheelchairs in and out of the car. He was my rock.

As a legacy for Andy, we set up a JustGiving page to get an all-terrain wheelchair specifically for children in the Yorkshire Dales National Park. We raised £16,000 and TerrainHopper donated a second chair. A different company gifted us another three chairs and it took off from there. So, we turned my blog, *Access the Dales*, into a charity, and now we have six hubs in the Dales where people can borrow wheelchairs. I cry every time I see a picture of somebody out using the chair because I know that that is changing their lives.

Andy's friend John and I began to put on days when people can come with their own wheelchairs and join us for a walk. For instance, we ran a day out at Ingleborough National Nature Reserve for people with visual impairments and there was a lady who had no vision whatsoever. She 'saw' the scenery through her own imagination and felt the wind on her face and heard the sounds of nature. And it was just wonderful to listen to her. She couldn't thank us enough for taking her on this journey.

Now we're working on how we can provide access to the countryside for people with all kinds of disability and it's just such an exciting journey. I was on the ITV *Tonight* programme last night and 15 people booked their wheelchairs within half an hour of the programme finishing.

Rhiane: That's wonderful! How do you see your work developing?

Debbie: We are having an impact now. I was appointed by the Cabinet Office as their Disability and Access Ambassador for the countryside, helping ministers to understand the lack of access and what people are doing around the country.

Wonderful things are happening but there's no cohesion. I'm campaigning now to have statutory guidelines for what makes an easy access route, for example – what is suitable for all, suitable for some and suitable for many. I was also awarded a Points of Light award by the prime minister for everything that I'm doing as a volunteer. It keeps me busy!

I'm working with the RSPB, who are trying to make a nature reserve at Haweswater more accessible and I've just finished a project with the Eden River Trust, so now a wheelchair user can get on the train and then have a lovely walk down the River Eden. And I am involved with Natural England and developing The Countryside Code so that it connects with people with disabilities.

Sometimes I go to bed at night, and I think, *Little old me has just had a meeting with the bigwigs from Natural England and the minister at Westminster.* It's unreal. I cannot believe that I've got this far. And it is an absolute passion.

Rhiane: How do you encourage ordinary people to participate in the outdoors?

Debbie: I look at it like this: we all have our own Everest, and it might be a small walk, or climbing a mountain. Having that 'I can do it' moment is so special. Especially after the pandemic: for lots of vulnerable people and people with long-term illness who have been shielding for so long, a sense of social isolation has become the norm for many. It's a mental health issue, getting people outside again, persuading them that it's safe to do so.

I feel very privileged in the fact that I know there are national parks, and I can visualise where they are in my mind map. But some people don't know what a national park is. Some people would not have a clue.

On the other hand, I'm so grateful for the pandemic because it gave me really precious time with Andy. If we hadn't been forced to stay together at home, I'd have been off doing this and that. We were spotting wildflowers that we'd never seen before, and we asked each other, 'Have they always been there? Or have we been in too much of a rush to notice them?'

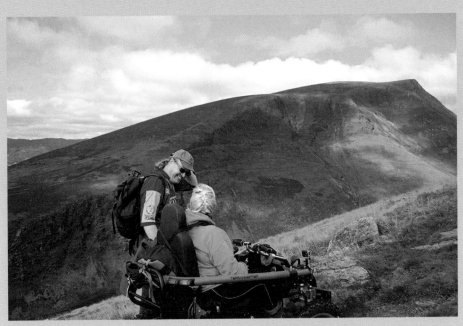

➡ Having that 'I can do it' moment is so special.

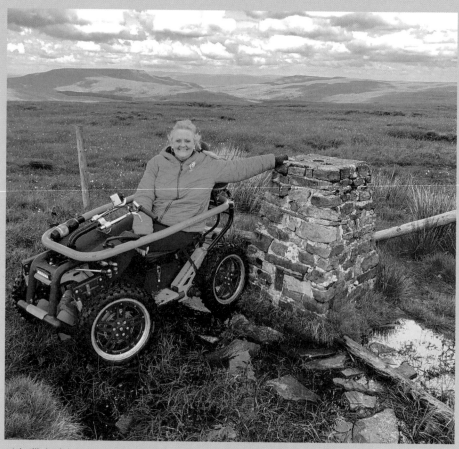

➡ I still don't know where I can go on my mobility scooter. Information is vital.

Rhiane: So you've had like all these achievements now and you're working with some big organisations, really making an impact. What has been the pivotal moment for you?

Debbie: I think the continuing challenge is finding out information. You know I would say I'm quite a confident person and I'm travelling around on my own now. But I'm fearful. I've bought a camper van, which is a big moment in my life, but then I take my camper van somewhere and I still don't know where I can go for a walk.

The national parks have used this title 'Miles Without Stiles' but there is no cohesion as to what standards they're using. So, what may be considered an easy access route for one national park isn't comparable with what an easy access walk is in another. I'm talking to the minister about how we can get statutory guidelines.

And then there's getting the information about all the good work that's happening around the countryside out there so that, within three or four clicks, people know where they can go to enjoy a route with their mobility scooter.

66
KEEP GOING, EVEN IF IT'S SPENDING JUST TEN MINUTES IN YOUR GARDEN OR IN A PARK. FIND SOME GREEN SPACE.
99

Rhiane: What did the minister say about this?

Debbie: He was amazed that it wasn't already like that. My term of office is for three years and if it's the only thing I achieve in those three years, I'll feel satisfied that I've done something to serve the community of disabled people and helped them to get outside.

Rhiane: You should be recognised for this work, be honoured.

Debbie: Honestly, those kind of things don't bother me. It's not a glory thing. It's that I can't believe that we're in the 21st century and there are people who can't get outside because they've got a disability. I just find that so sickening and sad. So, if by what I'm doing I can inspire people, raise aspirations and make a difference at a strategic level, I'll go and join Andy up on the mountain one day and say, 'We did it, kid, we did it!'

Rhiane: Finally, what would you say to somebody who wants to find their feet in the outdoors?

Debbie: Keep going, even if it's spending just ten minutes in your garden or in a park. Find some green space. You know, if you can take your shoes and socks off and put your feet on the ground and just connect with Mother Nature, you will feel immediately good. You will. And that moment of feeling good, bottle it and use it as your energy to go a little bit further afield and explore what is just beyond the boundaries of your home.

Rhiane: That's beautiful, Debbie. Andy would be very, very proud!

EPILOGUE

TIME TO GET OUT THERE

I hope you have enjoyed reading this book as much as I have writing it! Putting all this information and all these individual stories together has been a real adventure . I feel very fortunate to have had this chance to look back over my life and my journey since those first steps into the wilderness. There is so much useful stuff here, so many great women I've met, and fantastic hikes completed, that I am quite amazed at how over the last five years I have completely transformed the way I live. Now my passion has become my career and I couldn't be happier.

It makes me realise how different my life could have been if I hadn't decided to take up hiking. Everything I have achieved since then – from leading exploratory trips to Morocco and Ghana and TV work, to being invited to Buckingham Palace to talk about BGH – has stemmed from that single decision. But it's not just my journey in this book, there are lots of other fantastic women who have found their feet in the outdoors. I really hope that the wealth of knowledge and experience they have been generous enough to share have given you loads of ideas of how you too can begin your own adventure.

I also hope you have found that taking your first steps into the outdoors and into a more relaxed, fitter and environmentally aware future is easier than you thought when you first picked up this book. Though the range of equipment (and all the associated advertising!) can make it seem expensive and complicated to take part in outdoor activities, that couldn't be further from the truth. Still wondering where to start? Then pull on your trainers and head to your local park, and go further than you have done before. Soon, you'll find that breathing fresher air, noticing the variety of trees, plants and wild animals, and the steady rhythm of your steps will have a calming effect.

If you begin to crave a wilder environment, longer hikes and the kind of drop-dead-gorgeous views you see on your friend's social media, then you have all the advice you need between these pages to start striking out further afield. The world is yours for the taking, you just have to reach out, and of course, put one foot in front of the other!

My story and those of the other women I interviewed demonstrate that it is possible to radically change your life through embracing the outdoors. What's more, race, age and disability need not prevent you from adventuring – I hope that our honest discussion of the barriers we have worked around (and sometimes smashed down!) show that it is possible for everyone to access the natural environment. THE countryside, is YOUR countryside. Rural areas do not simply belong to the people who live in them. Get out there and enjoy it!

INDEX

ABOUT THE AUTHOR

Rhiane Fatinikun MBE is an adventurer, TV presenter and advocate who champions the positive impact of the outdoors on mental health, and is committed to breaking down the barriers that restrict marginalised communities from accessing open spaces.

In 2019 Rhiane founded the UK's largest Black female-led lifestyle and outdoor collective Black Girls Hike, formed in response to a lack of safe spaces for Black women in nature. Rhiane is also an Ambassador for the Wildlife Trusts and Mountain Training, and in recognition of her work she is a recipient of the RGS Geographical Award. Acknowledged as a Positive Role Model for Gender at the National Diversity Awards, listed as one of Forestry England's 10 most powerful women in nature, and named Campaigner of the Year by The Great Outdoors Awards, in 2024 Rhiane was awarded an MBE for services to nature and diversity.